DOCTOR, PLEASE HELP ME DIE

DOCTOR, PLEASE HELP ME DIE

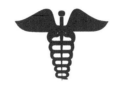

TOM PRESTON, MD

with

Janice Harper, PhD

iUniverse, Inc.
Bloomington

Doctor, Please Help Me Die

The following editions of Bible are used throughout the text, using abbreviations for King James Version (KJV), New King James Version (NKJV), New International Version (NIV), and English Standard Version (ESV)

iUniverse books may be ordered through booksellers or by contacting:

iUniverse
1663 Liberty Drive
Bloomington, IN 47403
www.iuniverse.com
1-800-Authors (1-800-288-4677)

ISBN: 978-1-4759-6379-3 (sc)
ISBN: 978-1-4759-6381-6 (e)
ISBN: 978-1-4759-6380-9 (dj)

Library of Congress Control Number: 2012924189

Printed in the United States of America

iUniverse rev. date: 1/10/2013

To Molly, Stephanie, and Hilary, without whom I would be lost.

Contents

Acknowledgments

Although the thesis of this book is the failure of many physicians to help their patients die peacefully, the greatest help I have had in writing it is the unswerving devotion of those physicians who have acted above and beyond common medical practice in honoring their patients' requests for aid in dying.

Some of these physicians I have known or at least met, and many I have never met but have known from their patients and the patients' families the eternal gratitude they have for the caring these physicians have shown.

I am indebted to Janice Harper, who is a medical anthropologist, for adding a cultural context to the history of assisted dying, for inserting humanity and fine writing to the manuscript, and for her encouragement in many ways.

And, of course, an author can never underestimate the support of family and friends, ever encouraging and supportive.

INTRODUCTION

IN THE FINAL BOOK of the Harry Potter series, a leading character is the recipient of a deadly magical curse. Realizing he has only a year left to live, he appeals to a friend and colleague to kill him. The friend responds that doing so might leave his own soul eternally damaged, to which the dying character replies, "You alone know whether it will harm your soul to help an old man avoid pain and humiliation. I ask this one great favor of you ... because death is coming for me."

Death comes for us all, and the desire to ease into that death is as ancient as humankind. Yet the topic is a troublesome one, because who among us has the power and knowledge to help us die best but those we entrust to heal us—our physicians? The very thought that our physicians might help us die is unsettling, because should they abuse that trust, the ramifications would be profound. Moreover, in the views of many, only divine intervention—rather than medical intervention—should determine our end.

As I show in the pages to follow, such belief assumes medical intervention does not already determine when and how we die, but medical intervention does indeed determine when and how we die. It not only extends life artificially and prevents natural death, but physicians routinely facilitate patients' deaths in complex and often unseen ways. Doctors passively encourage or facilitate death by providing or withholding treatments, making decisions about the type of care a patient will or won't receive, and otherwise intervening to prolong or terminate a patient's suffering.

And they do so both within and outside the law. Yet efforts to ease the laws that limit what physicians can and cannot do inevitably meet with considerable debate—and physicians themselves are often in the forefront of resisting the very laws that would enable them to help patients die with more compassion. The truth is, physician-assisted dying, or PAD, is an emotionally volatile topic that in recent years has become so politicized that even heads of state find themselves making public pronouncements on the topic. George W. Bush went so far as to fly back to Washington, DC, to sign a special bill blocking the removal of life support from Terri Schiavo. In France, President François Mitterrand made no secret of his intolerance for the legalization of PAD. But when his own death was near, President Mitterrand had a different view. Throughout his long political career, President Mitterrand had opposed "mercy killing," or any form of assisted death to end suffering. Having experienced firsthand the horrors of Nazi Germany as a POW, he viewed assisted death as a form of euthanasia and would not support its legalization. Perhaps his position was shaped, in part, by the secret he kept throughout his presidency, shared only with his personal physician—the French president was suffering from prostate cancer.

Mitterrand endured his suffering in silence for fifteen years, but when the disease had spread beyond his ability to conceal it and his death was close at hand, he requested that treatment stop. Following a lavish if not controversial last meal, in which he feasted on platters of oysters, foie gras, and capon before swallowing two or three yellow-throated, thumb-sized birds—bones, beak, and all[1]—President Mitterrand announced, "I'm eaten up inside."[2] Eight days later he was dead—from lack of food and medicine it was thought at the time—but the rumors that swirled for years have been confirmed: contrary to the position he had long held, the president had asked his physician to help him die.[3]

While Mitterrand's death may have been unusual for a head of state if he was helped by his physician, the idea that sometimes it is better to die quickly and in control of that death—rather than linger in pain and misery once impending death is certain—has troubled yet comforted humankind. The concept is troubling because to take death into one's hands implies a certain temerity—who dares suggest he or she knows better when and how to orchestrate the ending of a life? And the idea is comforting because the knowledge that once our life is ending it need not torture us provides a certain solace. It means that someone might be there to help us go gently into that good night.

Perhaps one of the most succinct dramatizations of this conflict between whether or not it is ever appropriate to help another die is in the 1948 movie *An Act of Murder*. Fredric March plays Calvin Cooke, an unforgiving judge who has no use for mercy when sentencing the convicted. In his view, the circumstances of a crime or the mental state of the perpetrator might be explanations, but they are never an excuse. The act itself is all that matters to him when it comes to passing judgment.

But circumstances force the judge to confront his own values when his wife is diagnosed with a painful terminal illness. In consultation with her physician, family friend Dr. Walter Morrison, Judge Cooke decides to conceal from the wife he so deeply loves the seriousness of her illness; in so doing, he hopes she will enjoy her final days untroubled by the knowledge her life is coming to an end. But the rapid progression of her disease brings such pain that before long, he realizes he cannot bear to see her suffer any longer. In desperation, as she naps in the passenger seat beside him, the judge leaps from the car and sends it rolling over an embankment, his sleeping wife unaware that she is plunging to her death.

The judge then finds himself back in his own courtroom, but this time as a defendant willing to accept his punishment. He unapologetically confesses his guilt, insisting he be judged just as dispassionately as he has passed judgment on so many others.

Having acted with the intent to kill, he could not in his own mind plead that there was any justification for his crime, even though his act was motivated by his love for his suffering wife and his desire to free her from an excruciating death.

As his attorney cross-examines his wife's physician, Dr. Morrison, on the witness stand, the judge is confident that though he seeks no mercy, his friend will speak to his good character and explain the motives to his crime. But speaking openly before the courtroom, the doctor takes another position altogether. Asked by the defense attorney if it was natural to want to end the pain of a loved one, the doctor hesitates before answering that yes, such a desire is natural. The presiding judge expresses his astonishment and presses the doctor for his views on "mercy killing." The doctor, who had empathized with his friend's desperate act, states that he opposes mercy killing.

"Under *any* circumstances?" the judge asks.

"Under any circumstances," the doctor answers, as the courtroom erupts into disapproving murmurs.

The defendant leaps to his feet in astonishment, asking his friend how he could possibly change his views. But the pounding of the gavel silences him. Later, in his cell, as the doctor visits his jailed friend of many years, the condemned man begs to know what happened.

The doctor explains to his incarcerated friend that scientists are hard at work in laboratories throughout the world, and what might be incurable one day could be curable the next. But such an answer does not satisfy the man whose wife was suffering; he responds that when he saw his wife sleeping peacefully by his side, he wanted to be sure she remained at peace and never knew pain again.

"I knew then," he tells his friend, the doctor, "I didn't want her to have pain ever again. I was sure it was the only thing to do. And I was right, Walter. I was right, wasn't I?"

As his question lingers, the scene draws to a close, the camera never turning to reveal the face or thoughts of the doctor who had made his position clear. He might understand, but he could not publicly support the act of mercy killing.

Dr. Morrison's views on mercy killing may or may not be shared with others, but he was clearly right about one thing—what was incurable in 1948 may well be curable today. Never before in the history of the world have people lived as long—or died as slowly. People suffering from illnesses and injuries that were once lethal may now live months or even years longer than they would have only a generation ago; though death will eventually come, its delay is a priceless gift.

But all too often, when survival has been extended through technology, the life a terminally ill person is left with is anything but rewarding. With death indefinitely delayed, the dying must often endure such lingering agony that a meaningful life is no longer possible. In these cases, death delayed becomes suffering prolonged. As we have gained greater control over the dying process through our increasing capacity to extend life and stave off death, our capacity to relinquish this control in order to stop extending life has become all the more challenging. With technology playing an ever-greater role in determining when and how we die, patients, families, and healers are faced with uncomfortable and painful choices. If someone chooses to end his suffering and die, should a physician have the right—or duty—to assist in that objective? And if so, what should be the physician's role in that objective?

The answers to these questions are never simple or easy, yet data increasingly demonstrate that, if suffering from a terminal illness for which there is no relief, most Americans would prefer a swift and natural death rather than have their suffering prolonged through artificial means.[4] But if so many Americans would elect to end their life if they were dying slowly and any sort of meaningful life was no longer possible, why has it been so difficult in the United States for patients to end their suffering if that is what the majority want?

The answer to that question is not necessarily what many think; in fact, while many groups have been outspoken in their opposition of assisted death for the terminally ill, another far more silent group may well prove to be the greatest obstacle to passing laws that would make it possible for the dying to die sooner rather than later. And that group is physicians, including some who themselves (discretely) engage in the practice of PAD.

The vocal objection that certain religious and political groups have voiced regarding death-with-dignity legislation is well known. Among those who oppose the legalization of abortion, any intervention that seeks to end a life, other than the execution of criminals—which "right-to-life" supporters almost always support—is considered interfering with God's design; the right-to-life argument is thus extended from the developing fetus to the dying, and any legislation or policy that would facilitate death is consequently opposed. Similarly, some disabled groups have been outspoken in their concerns that any sanction of assisted death could resurrect the horrors of Nazi Germany's policy of euthanasia, if the lives of the disabled became viewed as undesirable. These concerns are understandable, but as I show in the pages that follow, they are almost always based on inaccurate perceptions of whom death-with-dignity laws are aimed to help, and how they would actually be put into practice.

Perhaps least understood of all in the debates on whether or not dying people, their families, or physicians should have the right to control the end of life is the role that physicians themselves have quietly played by their failure to support the legalization of assisted death. Just as the fictional Dr. Morrison demonstrated when he turned against the friend whose actions he had privately condoned, even when doctors facilitate patient-controlled deaths in their medical practices, a large number of them have been conspicuous in their silence concerning laws that would permit them to legally help their patients die more naturally. Moreover, it is not necessarily fundamentalist religious views that have influenced the silence of these physicians. Instead, it is the less perceptible but more far-reaching philosophical foundations of the broader Judeo-Christian tradition and Western medical professional practices that have shaped how life, death, and suffering are understood in the Western world—and why so many physicians prefer to assist death covertly and without the law's permission. In *Doctor, Will You Help Me Die?* I explore this phenomenon of physician silence regarding physician-assisted death and show how physicians have variously approached the subject in policy and in practice.

The book begins with a historical and social overview of assisted death, suffering, and medical technology. By taking the position that assisted death is only justified when the patient is already dying, I show that using the word "suicide" to refer to physician-assisted death is misleading and inaccurate and should not be used. Instead, I suggest that assisted death is morally and socially appropriate in specific contexts. Moreover, I show that assisted death is consistent with modern medical practice, while further demonstrating how medical practice has both concealed and carried out the practice that so many physicians publicly resist.

I begin by examining the mythical and philosophical roots of assisted dying before moving on to the heartbreaking cases of Karen Ann Quinlan, Nancy Cruzan, and Terri Schiavo, women who each suffered irreversible brain damage and became propelled into the national spotlight as the courts, and a divided public, debated their end-of-life care.

I then show how popular culture has portrayed assisted death throughout history, suggesting that physicians have long played a role in delivering their patients to the grim reaper while remaining bit players in most fictional portrayals that place the responsibility for the act upon the dying themselves, if not their friends and families. In fiction, it seems, the doctor's role as benevolent healer remains unblemished by the discomforting act of mercy killing. Just as Dr. Morrison's face was never shown after his friend's beseeching question, "I was right, wasn't I?" in popular culture, the role of doctors in assisted death remains invisible. That is, until Dr. Kevorkian burst onto the scene with his death machines, the "Thanatron" and the "Mercitron."

But unlike Dr. Kevorkian, whose criteria for assisted death were loosely defined and open to interpretation, I take a different approach. Consistent with how the majority of Americans view assisted death as something they would choose only if they were dying and no cure was possible, I suggest that only in cases of terminal illness is physician-assisted death justified.

Jumping headlong into the political maelstrom of the volatile debates that have been associated with assisted death, I demonstrate how political and social groups have variously framed the issue of PAD as "killing," "murder," and "suicide." I refute such narrow interpretations and show how these explanatory models have been based on false premises while deliberately excluding critical evidence and legitimate perspectives regarding the legal and moral foundations of PAD.

To better understand where much of this thinking is coming from, I show how Greek and Roman mythology and the Bible provide an explanatory model for affliction as something willed by God or gods and remained outside the hands of mortals. Just as indigenous societies often explain illness or injury as caused by witchcraft or ancestral punishment, the view of affliction as a punishment has a long history in human medicine. But the Western concept of sin and salvation have uniquely shaped these notions of illness and divine intervention by entwining these ideas with an impression of the sanctity of life—something so sacred that regardless of how the sufferer experiences it, any living breath is regarded as a gift from God. And any act that might stop the breath is thus viewed as an unspeakable defiance of his will.

I then examine the organizational culture of Western medicine itself, beginning with a case study that shows the many ways physicians resist patient requests for help to die. I trace the roots of medical education and ethical oaths from ancient Greece to contemporary medical school training. Despite popular belief that the phrase in the Hippocratic Oath indicating the doctor "shall give no poison" means modern physicians must not help their patients die peacefully, I take a close look at the actual oath itself, and its many variations.

After discussing the ethical conflicts and constraints physicians face in their training and their practice, I turn to the organizational cultures of the medical profession itself, from the professional organizations that exercise ideological control over physicians and act as the public face of the profession, to the hospitals, clinics, and offices in which they work, where decision making is a social process involving multiple parties and interests, from families to administrators to third-party insurers. By exploring the patient/healer relationship and the historical and social roots of the concept of healing, I show how assisted death has been resisted by the medical profession, even though assisted death is consistent with the concept of healing and bringing an end to suffering.

I build on this argument by examining how technology has shaped human suffering by extending life and drastically changing the very nature of how we die. I suggest medical technology has made natural dying an exception rather than the norm, and, along with it, has changed how we conceptualize the body and its control. I follow with a discussion of how doctors themselves have been deceptive, resisting the legalization of PAD while at the same time practicing it routinely but covertly—by withdrawing life support, providing lethal dosages of morphine and other medications, and inducing unconsciousness before withholding food and water necessary to sustain life.

By examining how the taking of a life for greater good is made socially acceptable and practiced openly in some societies, I argue that despite the philosophical and cultural forces that have shaped resistance to assisted death in the United States, there remains great latitude in rethinking the concept. But as technology has removed death from life by making it more isolated from daily living and more remote from view, we understand it less.

As I elaborate on my explanation of how most people now die differently compared to just sixty years ago, I also point out that the rise of the hospice movement has also shaped how we view death. When the dying are removed from the control of the physician and the organizational culture of medicine and placed into a separate space for dying, hospice can provide an invaluable caregiving service. However, hospice care does not include aid in dying, nor do most hospices aid patients in obtaining physician-assisted dying.

By advocating a shift from physician-centered medicine to a meaningful patient-centered approach, I demonstrate how too much of what has been presented as patient-centered medicine has actually done more to benefit the physician than the patient.

In the final chapters, I discuss the legal and political debates that have distorted actual medical practice and been permeated by ideological viewpoints that represent a minority view in our nation, but have had disproportionate impact on medical care and policy. I suggest there is a "conspiracy of silence" surrounding the unspoken agreement among health-care providers of what to do or not do in efforts to alleviate suffering and hasten death. Drawing from the ideas presented in previous chapters, I analyze why it is preferable for some physicians to maintain the silent practice of assisted death while resisting the legalization of the practice. Nonetheless, I suggest physicians who will not assist their patients in dying are actually inflicting pain and suffering, and helping patients end their lives peacefully is as much a part of health-care delivery as is treating any ailment.

Finally, in a postscript, I provide recommendations for how patients can work effectively with their health-care providers and families to ensure their own deaths are as natural and comfortable as possible once the inevitable time has come and death is on its way.

One final thought before diving into the book. A number of different terms have been used, or misused, to characterize physician-assisted death, and the reader may be understandably confused. I use the term "medically managed dying" when a medical act such as removing a feeding tube or disconnecting a patient from a ventilator leads to the patient's death. "Physician-assisted dying" or "physician-assisted death" (both abbreviated as PAD) refer to providing dying patients a prescription or medication the patient can take to end his or her life. It does not refer to the physician injecting any lethal medication into a patient—that is euthanasia. I do not advocate euthanasia under any circumstances, and my book is not intended to be an argument in its support.

"Mercy killing" is another term generally used to refer to euthanasia, although it has also been used to refer to PAD. That term, I suggest, is thus problematic. Moreover, I see no value, yet considerable harm, in characterizing PAD as any form of "killing." Indeed, it is a central premise of my book that PAD is *not* a form of killing or murder, at least as we understand the concept morally, ethically, and legally, and I elaborate on my reasoning in this book.

"Physician-assisted suicide" refers to a patient taking the medication a physician has provided or prescribed, but as I explain, that term is also problematic because to end one's suffering when death is imminent is not the same as *choosing* to end life. When that end is inevitable, unavoidable, and imminent—but fraught with such physical suffering that the patients are forced to accept that undesired end sooner rather than unnaturally later—the dying do not "commit suicide." They want to live, not die. But if die they must, then they want to do so with dignity and grace. And they want to do so with the respect and acceptance of family, friends, physicians, and society.

This, then, is my case—as a physician and cardiologist who has cared for thousands of dying patients throughout my forty-year career—for why we as physicians have a responsibility to our patients to heal their end-of-life suffering as only we are able. And why we, as a society, have a responsibility to extend our compassion—and basic human rights—to the dying *even if to do so is discomforting and seemingly inconsistent with our own religious or moral views.*

In a nation founded on the separation of church and state, to allow a singular religious viewpoint to determine the medical care we may or may not receive is contrary to the very basis of democracy and decency in our modern but imperfect world. What follows is my argument for why every citizen who is dying ought to be extended an inalienable right to die peacefully, and why every physician has an ethical obligation to assist patients who want to exercise this right safely, securely, and painlessly.

Chapter 1
A Short History of the Right to Die

I F TO KILL IS a cruelty because it robs one of life, what does it mean to rob a person of death? Society has long grappled with the question of whether it is morally acceptable for physicians to end the suffering of someone who is dying. But I ask a different question here: Is it morally acceptable for physicians to refuse to do so? If a physician can ease a person's suffering and make his or her final moments of life endurable and peaceful by helping the patient die, is it wrong to refuse to do so? Could nonaction be a greater cruelty than action when someone's pain is agonizing and readily ended by medication or other help from his or her physician?

Consider the case of Heracles. Heracles, or Hercules as he is more commonly called, was the half-god son of Zeus and the beautiful, mortal Alcmene. Zeus endowed his son with superhuman strength, an attribute that made him a rather troublesome child but nevertheless enabled him to conquer pretty much any challenge he was presented. When Heracles found himself in a bit of a mess for slaughtering his family (his superhuman strength surpassed only by his superhuman temper, a temper brought on by madness inflicted by his vengeful stepmother, Hera), he was punished by having to endure a series of superhuman feats. He strangled a lion, traveled to hell and back, killed a multiheaded hydra monster, and accomplished several other highly unpleasant, dangerous, and seemingly impossible tasks that, through brute strength and unwavering persistence, he managed to pull off with seeming ease. But for all the painful trials Heracles had overcome, none was as great as enduring the horrific agony of death. Tricked into donning a beautiful cloak that had been soaked in a powerful poison that burned the flesh off anyone who wore it, Heracles screamed in agony the moment the lethal robe touched his skin. He flung off the robe, but alas, all his flesh came with it, skinning alive the man of superhuman strength. Suffering unbearable pain, the immortal god demanded his son help him die.

"You are asking me to be your murderer," the young man answered, refusing to comply with his father's dying command.

"No," Heracles replied, "I am not. I ask you to be my healer, the only physician who can cure my suffering."

But his son refused to help him. Powerless because the only healer who could help him refused to do so, Heracles was forced to die slowly and in great agony. Unable to withstand the pain any longer, he ordered his funeral pyre built. Once it was done, he threw himself into the flames to end the excruciating torture. To burn alive was preferable to the agony of suffering any longer.

Flash forward to the twentieth century, and a woman of ordinary strength confronts the pain of dying. "I am now about to make the great adventure," actress Clara Blandick wrote in 1962, when she was slowly dying with severe arthritis. "I cannot endure this agonizing pain any longer. It is all over my body. Neither can I face the impending blindness. I pray the Lord my soul to take. Amen." Setting her pen down, the eighty-two-year-old woman, immortalized thirty years earlier as "Auntie Em" in *The Wizard of Oz*, dressed in a beautiful blue gown with her hair perfectly set, lay down on her couch, and took an overdose of pills that her doctor had prescribed to treat her constant pain. She covered herself with a golden blanket and died, surrounded by her favorite photos and press clippings, commemorating a life well lived, with no regrets. Like Heracles, Clara Blandick didn't want to die, but neither did she want to endure a slow agony from severe arthritis that only death could cure.

Sophocles, writing twenty-five hundred years ago, was among the first to address this human tragedy through drama when he narrated the story of Heracles's death in the Athenian tragedy *The Women of Trachis*. Sophocles understood the desire of dying patients to end their suffering by ending life. "Best by far," he wrote, "when one has seen the light, is to go thither swiftly whence he came."[5]

Sophocles wasn't the only Greek tragedian who recorded the common sentiment. Aeschylus wrote, "Oh that in speed without pain and the slow bed of sickness death could come to us now."[6] Seneca, the Roman stoic, expanded on the theme. He wrote, "The wise man will consider it of no importance whether he causes his end or merely accepts it. … Dying early or late is of no relevance; dying well or ill is. To die well is to escape the danger of living ill."[7]

As these philosophers and dramatists understood, the desire to end suffering by dying quickly is eternal in the history of mankind. Yet the concept of suffering is inextricably woven into a tapestry of beliefs regarding humanity's relationship to the Divine, lacing together the medical and the religious as new technologies raise new questions concerning the changing cultural roles—and powers—of physicians.

A couple years ago I was talking to a legislator who was sponsoring a bill to ban physician aid in dying. I told him how, as a physician, I was distressed to see so much needless suffering at the end of life. He lurched toward me in his seat and asked, "What's wrong with suffering?" As he put it, the concept of needless suffering seemed not just incongruous but unbelievable. I had trouble even replying. Does anyone like to suffer? How could he think there isn't anything wrong with suffering?

To most people, such a question as the legislator posed might appear cruel, even sadistic. But I knew the argument well enough to recognize where he was going with his line of thought. The legislator was of the mindset that people have a duty to share the burden of Christ's suffering and that through suffering comes redemption. As the Catholic writer Joseph Sullivan said, "Suffering is almost the greatest gift of God's love."[8]

The concept of suffering to attain salvation can be traced to the apostle Paul and St. Augustine, who wrote about Christ's love for those who suffered and the need to accept one's suffering as a trial, just as Job suffered his afflictions in silence knowing his Lord would not forsake him. But it has not been until recent years that the concept of suffering has been embraced by the far right as a justification for a variety of deprivations and social sacrifices. It is little wonder, then, that the concept of suffering as divine has been used to justify refusing aid to the dying in the form of physician-assisted death.

What may be surprising, however, is that this very same argument arose over whether women should have anesthesia for childbirth. In yet another battlefield for the will of God, during the mid-nineteenth century, when chloroform was introduced as an anesthesia during childbirth, many physicians and clergy argued that to interfere with the pain of childbirth would be a violation of God's will. They based their argument on the belief that after the fall of the first parents, Adam and Eve, God cast a primeval curse upon humanity, proclaiming, "in sorrow thou shalt bring forth children" (Genesis 3:16). The dispute over whether women should have pain relief in childbirth continued for several years, and effectively ended in 1853 when Queen Victoria took chloroform during the birth of her eighth child.[9]

Lest the reader think the nineteenth-century belief that suffering is divine has no influence on the practice of modern secular medicine, consider the work of President George W. Bush's Council on Bioethics. The council, established on November 28, 2001, by Executive Order 13237, was directed to "advise the president on bioethical issues that may emerge as a consequence of advances in biomedical science and technology." The council's report stated, "Yet human pain, while possibly more frequent and intense than animals', is also privileged in a way that that of animals never can be: our suffering, and ours alone, may perhaps be redeemed."[10]

Moreover, this view is not limited to conservative Christians; Catholicism embraces a similar perspective on the concept of suffering. For example, on July 25, 2011, at a Kansas City conference on end-of-life care, Cardinal Burke, prefect of the Apostolic Signatura, said, "No matter how much a life is diminished, no matter what suffering the person is undergoing, that life demands the greatest respect and care. It's never right to snuff out a life because it's in some way under heavy burden."[11]

And although some Catholic teaching does support stopping treatment that is "extraordinary" or "disproportionate" in prolonging meaningless and burdensome life, under the most orthodox teaching it is never allowable to end life in order to minimize suffering, even when the patient is days or weeks from dying.

Although many people of faith support both medically managed dying and physician aid in dying, the most ardent opponents come from the ranks of those with strong convictions based on religious tenets, predominantly self-described advocates of what is commonly termed a "right to life." In many surveys of demographics, attitudes, and preferences of voters, the element most closely correlated with opposition to physician aid in dying is religiosity, as measured by attendance at religious services and parameters pointing to fundamentalist religious beliefs. Surveys of physicians in several states, and nationally, have found the same, with a consistent core of 25–30 percent of physicians saying that physician aid in dying is unacceptable under any conditions.

Because the suffering of extended, unnatural dying is a new phenomenon, as I will show, society is floundering mightily in dealing with it. We still see—and label—life-ending acts in the old way, which is to say as killing. And yet, in virtually all societies, not all lives are sanctified, with the exception of Buddhist teachings, which hold that all life is sacred, yet nonetheless conclude that assisted death *can* be justified.

For all the resistance to physician aid in dying, there is an equally strong—indeed, far stronger—social tide toward embracing it. Today, everyone old enough to have watched a loved one die—a family member, friend, or even a casual acquaintance—knows the all-too-common and persistent agonies of dying. And physicians, whose stock in trade is to observe, know only too well the rigors of dying. For many patients, modern medical methods—in particular good comfort care with painkillers and treatments for other symptoms—can provide relatively peaceful ends. In these cases, there is no need for assisted death; it will come gently and in its own time.

But for those modern medicine fails, no amount of comfort care can alleviate the agonies of death. Far worse, while modern medicine may fail to help some people, it may instead *extend* the agonies of death by artificially extending life. And running the treacherous rapids of the dying process is not something anyone would wish for oneself or for a loved one. Yet it is indeed an issue that humanity has long grappled with, perhaps no better summed up than in six simple words from Shakespeare, famously penned in *Hamlet*: "To be, or not to be, that is the question."

Of course the existential struggle that the bard referred to spoke more to the sufferings of heartache and calamity than the ravages of dying flesh, yet the question of whether one ought to "take arms against one's troubles" when those troubles be the agonies of death have long bemused audiences through literature and theater, particularly throughout the twentieth century, when modern medicine made it possible to diagnose terminal illnesses at an early stage, prolong the lives of the dying, and discretely and painlessly end suffering with medicine.

Karen Ann Quinlan and Nancy Cruzan

Leaping forward several hundred years, we find the troublesome issue no more resolved than it was in antiquity, much less during Shakespeare's time. The emotionally evocative issue of whether a person should be allowed to die became a powerful social concern in the mid-1970s when the celebrated case of a young woman brought to public light what it means to keep someone alive through life support.

In 1975, Karen Ann Quinlan was a twenty-one-year-old woman who fasted for two days and then went to a party, where she ingested a combination of drugs and alcohol. By the end of the evening she had fallen into an irreversible coma, eventually deteriorating to a persistent vegetative state with no possible hope for recovery. When it was clear their daughter would never regain consciousness, her parents requested the hospital disconnect her life support and allow her to die. The hospital refused, so the Quinlan family—who were devout Roman Catholics—took their plea to the courts, asking that they be allowed to disconnect their daughter from the respirator.

But the Chancery Court denied the Quinlans' request, ruling that the question of whether to stop life support was a medical and not a judicial concern. The court then went one step further and took away any rights the parents had to make medical decisions regarding their daughter's care on the grounds that they were allegedly too traumatized to make reasoned judgments. With that decision, the case quickly turned from a tragic but private family matter to a sensationalized legal and social debate that made daily newspaper headlines and became fodder for nightly talk shows. Never before had the question of what it means to extend life through technology been so openly discussed, and now it was front-page news.

"The case was the first one to draw the attention of the country and the courts to the problem of being a prisoner in a helpless body, supported only by medical technology," John Fletcher, director of the Center for Medical Bioethics at the University of

Virginia noted.[12] "Death is not something that just happens to most people. Nowadays it's death by decision," he added. "Every one of those decisions is a direct descendant of the Quinlan decision."

After the Chancery Court ruling, the Quinlans took their case to the New Jersey Supreme Court, which reversed the Chancery Court's decision and ruled that Ms. Quinlan be disconnected from all life support. In reaching its decision, the court noted that were she competent to make the decision, Karen Ann Quinlan would have the right to decide for herself whether or not to sustain her life through medical technology, even if doing so led to her death.[13]

Following the State Supreme Court ruling, Ms. Quinlan was disconnected from life support, with the exception of continued feeding. But despite expectations that she would die quickly once disconnected, she lived for another ten years before finally succumbing to pneumonia in a nursing home in 1985.[14]

Meanwhile, another young woman, a once-lively twenty-five-year-old reduced to a vegetative state following a car accident in 1983, lay in a coma. Nancy Cruzan was a young Missouri woman whose parents fought for years, like the Quinlans, for their daughter to be allowed to die. When the Missouri Supreme Court ruled that the state's right to preserve life was absolute and her parents could not remove her feeding tube, her family took the case to the US Supreme Court.

Although the court upheld the lower court's ruling in respect to Ms. Cruzan, it made a finding that continues to shape patients' rights in respect to treatment and death. The US Supreme Court ruled that people who have the capacity to reason and make their own decisions *do* have the constitutional right to refuse treatment. Although that 1990 ruling did not help their daughter, the Cruzans found further evidence shortly after that their daughter had told others that she would not want to be kept alive artificially if she were ever in such a state. After presenting their new evidence to the state, the state of Missouri allowed the

Cruzans to disconnect their daughter's feeding tube. After nearly eight years of unconsciousness and without the capacity to think, Nancy Cruzan died peacefully at the age of thirty-three.

The Right to Die on Stage and Screen

The public display of these families' private torment in making the decision to allow their daughters to die had a deep effect on American society. It is therefore little wonder that the issue of death with dignity became increasingly explored in popular culture. Among the most successful of these explorations was Brian Clark's play *Whose Life Is It Anyway?* Written three years prior to the Quinlan case, the play wasn't produced until after the Quinlan case had made headlines, but it proved so popular that several adaptations followed. Most popular was the 1981 movie adaptation starring Richard Dreyfus as a brilliant young sculptor who is in a terrible car accident. The accident leaves him a quadriplegic dependent upon dialysis to live, confining him to hospital care for the rest of his life.

Unlike Karen Ann Quinlan, who was unaware of the fierce battle her tortured life had provoked, the fictional Ken Harrison is fully aware of his condition. After six months of lying motionless in his hospital bed, joking with the nursing staff, and appearing every bit the "life of the infirmary party," he summons his lawyer and tells him he would like to be discharged from the hospital to return home to die a natural death.

In the scenes that follow, the patient is trapped not only in a body that no longer functions but in a battle with his own physician, played by John Cassavetes, who holds strong views about the sanctity of life and his responsibility to preserve it. When one of his physicians makes it clear to Harrison that it is against her morals to assist him, Harrison quickly points out that her morals are considered better than his own only because she has more power than he has. Indeed, power is at the heart of the patient's struggle to make his own decisions concerning his body, as he is subjected to the daily indignities of being powerless to control his body and his medical care, while eventually appealing to the power of the courts to give him permission to make his own health-care decisions—even if doing so means he will die.

Harrison explains to the court that he does not want to die, but instead feels as if he is already dead; unable to work as an artist or live as a man, his life holds no more meaning. Describing the torment of an imagination that has been imprisoned in a useless body, Harrison considers what madness he might endure if the judge were to return in another five years to see what his lifeless life has done to that mind. The patient concludes that he is not asking anyone to commit an act of violence but to merely discharge him from the hospital. When Harrison suggests that to do otherwise would be an act of cruelty, the judge counters that it could be equally cruel not to save people's lives.

"No," Harrison responds, "because the cruelty is not a question of saving someone's life or letting him die. The cruelty is that the choice is removed from the person concerned."

Ultimately, the judge reluctantly sides with Harrison and agrees that if he does not want further medical intervention, a patient has the right to deny the treatment, citing the case of Karen Ann Quinlan. Once free to be discharged, his physician softens. He suggests to Harrison that to ensure his comfort, he remain in the hospital to die, and that no further life support would be provided unless he were to change his mind.

Harrison is tucked into bed, the curtains to his room are closed, and as is typical of movies featuring "mercy killing" or right-to-die issues—indeed, as is typical of real-life physician care—the physicians depart from the pending death scene, leaving their patient to die alone.

A similar theme would be repeated twenty-five years later in Clint Eastwood's 2004 Academy Award–winning film *Million Dollar Baby*. Hillary Swank plays a young boxer who is left a quadriplegic following a fight, confined to an extended-care facility where she is tied to a latticework of technology, a respirator helping her breathe twenty-four hours a day, and a wall of monitors constantly measuring the unseen movements beneath her unmovable flesh.

After losing her leg to gangrene and realizing the permanency of her injuries, she declares her desire to die and makes several futile attempts to end her own life, but each time a nurse arrives to stop her. The resistance of the medical staff to their patient's decision is as unmistakable as it is understated. Every effort the patient makes to exert what little power she has to end her life leads to increasing efforts by hospital staff to take away that power. The doctors and nurses are presented as diligent caregivers who view their roles as preservers of life, not angels of death. But they remain bit players in the film, and by the film's final scenes, they are offstage altogether as the patient turns to her trainer and friend, played by Clint Eastwood, and asks him to help her die.

There is no dramatic courtroom scene or speech to explain why dying would be preferable to living, other than a brief consultation Eastwood's character has with a priest who says it would be a sin for him to carry out the task of helping his friend die. There is no battle with administrators, no trial or tribunal to move the conflict from the private to social arena. It is sufficient that she states she wants to die while she can still hear the applause of the crowd cheering for her when she was a champion in the ring. By presenting the moral dilemma the main characters face as a private, individual matter, the dilemma remains shrouded in secrecy with its resolution to be made in silence. It is no wonder that the final scenes are filmed in near darkness, the only illumination cast upon the actors and the monitors that define their terrible dilemma.

Yet unlike *Whose Life Is It Anyway?*, where the central question was the right to refuse treatment and end one's own life, like 1948's *An Act of Murder*, *Million Dollar Baby* leaves the audience pondering the question: Is it ever appropriate to take someone else's life? A significant difference between these two films, however, illuminates a crucial moral distinction many make in determining under what conditions assisted death is appropriate.

In 1948's *An Act of Murder*, the protagonist is on trial for taking the life of a woman who was dying, whereas in 2004's *Million Dollar Baby*, the patient was not dying; like Ken Harrison in *Whose Life Is It Anyway?*, she was disabled. The issue of assisted death had moved from helping the dying to die a better death to helping the disabled die a premature death. And with that shift came an even more polarized debate, one that hit the front page once again, but this time under the guise of a self-appointed "Dr. Death."

Enter Jack Kevorkian

Jack Kevorkian (1928–2011) was a renegade pathologist who had long battled conventional medical thinking. Early in his career, he advocated using prisoners for medical experiments in lieu of execution, and after experimenting on his own staff, he suggested blood from corpses could be transfused into the living. Such ideas quickly estranged him from the mainstream medical community and limited his career to part-time pathology jobs. Kevorkian's fascination with the dead extended to his personal life as well; in his spare time he painted macabre scenes of severed limbs and heads, which were often painted in blood or framed in blood-soaked wood.

Kevorkian's interest in death and poking a finger in the eye of authority brought him national attention beginning in 1987, when he tried to advertise in local Detroit newspapers for "death consulting." Although the newspapers refused to print the ads, Kevorkian soon encountered an ad someone else had placed in local newspapers—a request by a young quadriplegic man for a physician to help him die.

David Rivlin was twenty years old when a 1971 bodysurfing accident left him a quadriplegic with limited movement of his arms. But when an operation in 1986 left him unable to move even those—or to breathe voluntarily without the assistance of a respirator—he decided to end his life.

"It's not that I welcome death," he told *People* magazine. "It's just that I welcome it over life."[15] When Kevorkian heard of Rivlin's desire to end his life, he set about building a machine that would help him do so. When he was done, Kevorkian's first "suicide machine," which he termed the Thanatron, was ready for use. It would enable a person, even if paralyzed, to release a sedative that would render him or her unconscious before releasing a second lethal dose of medication that would stop the heart.

But when Kevorkian presented his device to Rivlin, the suffering man rejected it. "When people talk about abortion, they debate over when life begins," Rivlin said, explaining his desire to die. "For me the question was, 'When did death begin?' It began with the vent."[16]

"The vent" was the respirator that kept him alive, and Rivlin was not asking anyone to help him commit suicide, as Dr. Kevorkian offered, but to merely sedate him and remove the tube.

Rivlin was seeking what some physicians and medical ethicists term "passive euthanasia," which is the removal of life support so that natural death can occur. Rivlin's plea for help, which he eventually took to the courts, was a real-life imitation of fictional Ken Harrison's plea to be released from the hospital and allowed to die. When the court granted Rivlin's request, noting it was legal to refuse medical treatment, the quadriplegic man went home where, surrounded by friends and family, a physician sedated him and then removed the respirator that was keeping him breathing. Within a half hour he died, peacefully and painlessly.

As for Kevorkian, rejected by David Rivlin, he was left with his suicide machine. Although his efforts to advertise his services in death consulting had failed, a friend published an article about his machine and his interest in helping people to die, and soon Kevorkian was flooded with interest.[17] And he got his opportunity to put his machine to use when fifty-four-year-old Janet Adkins read one of his ads and contacted him to ask if he would help her die. Janet Adkins was a school teacher in Oregon who had been diagnosed the prior year with early onset Alzheimer's disease. She remained active, but as her memory impairment increased, she decided to end her life before she was completely disabled—and before she was considered too incompetent to make such a decision.

The story of Jack Kevorkian's meeting with Janet Adkins is well known. After he helped Ms. Adkins die in the back of his VW van, the part-time pathologist—who hadn't treated any living patients since medical school—went on to assist approximately 130 other people in ending their lives. As reporters flocked around the once-obscure laboratory doctor, Kevorkian battled the judicial system in a series of celebrated prosecutions that cost him his medical license and eventually led to his eight-year imprisonment in 1997 for second-degree murder when he was filmed on *Sixty Minutes* injecting lethal drugs into a fifty-two-year-old man with Lou Gehrig's disease (ALS).

Kevorkian's flagrant defiance of the medical and judicial systems brought so much attention to the issue of assisted death that laws controlling physician-assisted dying—and laws permitting it—were rapidly enacted, beginning with Michigan making assisted suicide a crime shortly after Kevorkian announced that he had helped Janet Adkins die. By the time he was imprisoned in 1997, Adkins's home state of Oregon passed the Death with Dignity Act, permitting doctors to prescribe medications to help people die, which was subsequently upheld by the US Supreme Court in 2006, making PAD a reality in those states that permitted it.

In the years between Kevorkian's first assisted death and his imprisonment, however, his actions colored nearly every American's view of assisted death as the testimonials of suffering patients made it clear that there was a real public interest in helping some suffering people die. Of equal concern to the public interest was safeguarding the rights of those who could potentially be abused by indiscriminate practitioners of assisted death, which Kevorkian increasingly appeared to be, as details of his "patients" came to light.

It turned out that Janet Adkins not only was *not* terminally ill, she was not at all physically impaired—she had played a rigorous game of tennis just days before her death. Even more disconcerting was that, although she was physically strong, she may have lacked the mental capacity to make such a monumental decision. As details were revealed about Janet Adkins's death and the deaths of others Kevorkian assisted, the question of just how candidates for assisted death were selected by the man who became known as "Dr. Death" became a legitimate concern. By the time he was sentenced to ten to twenty-five years in prison for manslaughter, it was revealed that of forty-seven cases of death Jack Kevorkian assisted, seventeen could have lived indefinitely; twenty-eight (60 percent) were not terminally ill, and thirteen people had no complaints of pain.[18] Three years later, a more comprehensive study by the *New England Journal of Medicine* found that only twelve were terminally ill, and autopsies revealed that five had nothing physically wrong with them. Divorced, widowed, or never-married people were disproportionately represented among his assisted suicides, suggesting those with less social support were more likely to seek him out, and although most people who receive assistance with their death are terminally ill men older than sixty-five, almost three-quarters of Kevorkian's assisted deaths were of women, and they very often expressed fear of "being a burden" to others.[19]

For example, the second woman Jack Kevorkian helped die was a forty-six-year-old single mother who was falsely diagnosed with multiple sclerosis. Her autopsy revealed that she did not have the disease after all and that her body was covered with bedsores, indicating that whatever was wrong with her, she was not receiving adequate care. In one case, Kevorkian helped with the suicide of a woman who complained of severe pelvic pain. It not only turned out that she had nothing wrong with her physically; she had a history of mental illness and depression and was abusing medications that may have increased her suicidal impulses.[20]

When an elderly woman who was in pain from severe arthritis and had had both legs amputated appealed to Dr. Kevorkian for help, he publicly said he would help her die if pain specialists did not come forward to help her. His appeal resonated with the public because one of the most compelling arguments for PAD is to end intolerable suffering and pain. But when at least seven pain specialists contacted him, none were put in contact with the suffering woman before Dr. Kevorkian helped her commit suicide.[21] Because palliative care could have enabled her to live a longer, more rewarding life, and she was denied that opportunity through Kevorkian's actions, the arguments of those who condemned the polarizing figure, who had become a powerful but faulty symbol for physician-assisted dying, were all the more supported.

While these statistics are grim reminders of how easily an alleged "lone maverick" can abuse his power when operating outside the law, the human stories behind the statistics are stark reminders that without clear guidelines, assisted death could be practiced to the detriment of some whose lives can and should be saved—while also undermining public support for legal assisted dying for those whose lives cannot be saved and who seek peaceful dying.

In short, Kevorkian did more than anyone before him, including Karen Ann Quinlan and Nancy Cruzan for bringing the need for assisted death to the American dinner table. But few did more to illuminate just how troubling PAD could be without safeguards and scrutiny. Kevorkian wasn't just helping the dying die more dignified deaths, he was helping the depressed, the damaged, and the diseased choose death instead of life when a better life might have been within their reach all along, had Kevorkian not come knocking. It is little wonder then, that just as he brought the issue of PAD to light and raised awareness, he polarized the populace on the issue, enabling each side to gain confidence that the battle was decided in its favor when, in fact, the battle had just begun.

The Case of Terry Schiavo and the
Politicization of Death with Dignity

If Kevorkian brought the issue of PAD to the kitchen table, it was Terry Schiavo who brought it to the podium. To show just how deeply politics and the law can get in the matter of how we die, nothing can compare to the case of Terry Schiavo. Terry Schiavo was twenty-six years old when she collapsed from cardiac arrest in 1990 at her condominium in Florida that she shared with her husband, Michael Schiavo. Although she was revived by paramedics, she suffered irreversible brain damage from lack of oxygen to her brain and could not even swallow enough food or water to sustain her life. Her prognosis was dire: she was in a persistent vegetative state with no chance of recovery.

Over the next several years, Ms. Schiavo remained in hospice care, where she was fed through a feeding tube but in all probability was unable to communicate, respond to stimuli, or even be aware of visitors to her bedside. Although she did not have an advance directive indicating what she would want done under the circumstances, in 1998 her husband petitioned the court to remove her feeding tube. But her parents wanted her kept alive, and a fierce battle between the once-amicable parties ensued, leading to a hotly debated national debate on whether she should be kept alive through life support when there was no evidence she was even conscious of her own life.

As her parents and husband battled over whether to keep her alive or allow her to die, Terri Schiavo's case was appealed fourteen times, with her feeding tube removed and reinserted again and again as court after court reversed prior rulings. The case became so politicized by "right-to-life" advocates that Florida Governor Jeb Bush and even his brother President George Bush signed executive orders overturning court rulings and mandating she be kept alive. Ultimately, in a standoff that pitted the local police against the national guard, the governor backed down, and the feeding tube was removed on March 18, 2005. On March 31, 2005, Terri Schiavo died.

The case of Terri Schiavo presented an important point of departure from earlier cases regarding extending life support. In the case of Karen Ann Quinlan, her parents wanted to disconnect her from a respirator that was *believed* to be keeping her alive (the fact that she continued to live after it was disconnected surprised her medical team). In the case of Terri Schiavo, her husband wanted her disconnected from a feeding tube that was, indisputably, keeping her alive. Thus it could be argued that removal of a feeding tube was a step beyond the case of Karen Quinlan, whose family kept her connected to her feeding tube. But in both cases, the primary question before the courts was whether family had the right to disconnect life-sustaining technology. What made the Schiavo case so much different, however, was the politicization of the issue as her life became a symbol not just for end-of-life debates but for political debates extending to conservative and religious political campaigns for elected office.

Days after her death, and amid the fury over whether Ms. Schiavo had a "right to life"—a term that was quickly used to characterize the debate on a topic that in earlier years would have been characterized as a "right to death with dignity" issue—a memo surfaced that had been written by the legal counsel for a Florida Republican senator. The memo characterized the conflict as "a great political issue" that could damage the Democratic Party, and "excite" the pro-life base that sought to overturn abortion. By linking assisted death with abortion, this sector hoped to make Terry Schiavo a political symbol that had little or nothing to do with end-of-life care and everything to do with a declared war upon "liberals" and the desire for conservative control over the legislature. The memo even went so far as to compare Ms. Schiavo's civil rights to those of Ted Bundy, suggesting that the serial killer's life was granted greater social protections than the brain-damaged woman's.[22] But the publication of the memo backfired when the blatant exploitation of such a tragic personal issue for political gain was no longer plausibly deniable.

Thus the issue of death with dignity that Kevorkian had so flagrantly turned into a macabre spectacle had once again been perverted. Assisted death was turned into partisan party politics, framed as a right-to-life issue that would become linked to abortion, religious fundamentalism, and conservative political agendas. How people really felt about whether to consider assisted death in their own or their loved ones' lives was less the issue than where you stood on the issue of assisted death. More and more it reflected not your views on medical care, suffering, or death but which political party you supported. And that factor, more than any other, determined how the public discussed the issue. How physicians approached the matter, however, was shaped by more complex political and religious factors than those the general public considered. But before delving into the standpoint of physicians, let us first look at how the public framed the issue in the wake of Terri Schiavo's life and death.

CHAPTER 2
FRAMING THE ISSUE

I N THE AFTERMATH OF Terri Schiavo's public life and death, it is little surprise that how we die not only became a religious issue for many Americans, but it also became a deeply political one. Whereas the cases of Karen Ann Quinlan and Nancy Cruzan were debated in the courts, the fate of Terri Schiavo went far beyond the courts, involving the highest levels of the US legislature and even the executive office of the president of the United States. In the aftermath of Jack Kevorkian and Terri Schiavo, virtually all states in the nation now have laws allowing or disallowing physician aid in dying. Like it or not, how we die is now very much a matter of civic action through the political process. And that means how we die is not necessarily as important to social policy as how we *speak of* dying.

Those who debate the topic of physician-assisted dying (PAD) understand the power of persuasion that comes of how an issue is framed. As we know, politics is the art of persuasion. The ancient Greeks called it rhetoric, or the art of speaking effectively regardless of the issue being discussed. Today the more popular buzzword is "framing," which means not so much arguing effectively as positioning the argument in terms favorable to your cause. Framing operates by taking seemingly disparate ideas and framing them within a single but broader concept, so our minds begin to discern patterns that we might not otherwise recognize.

For example, when the tobacco industry wanted to expand from an exclusively male market to include women, it promoted an ad campaign that associated smoking with freedom, liberation, and independence. Although the health hazards of smoking were just beginning to be recognized, as the women's movement brought issues of equality and independence to the public's mind, it wasn't long before many women responded to the cigarette ads and felt they too had a "right" to smoke. Despite the fact that cigarette smoking is highly addictive and any association with liberation or freedom is rather ironic, at an emotional level the framing of these two disparate concepts—smoking and freedom—worked. In no time at all, women took up smoking in numbers to equal those of men.

Politicians well understand, just as advertising executives do, that how an issue is framed will shape how it is perceived. By framing an issue in a manner that persuades the listener to share the *perceptions* of the speaker, it is much easier to persuade the listener to share the *position* of the speaker as well.

How then has the framing of the issue of assisted death changed over time? Let us begin with Heracles's plea for his son to help him die, and his son's refusal to do so on the grounds that it would constitute "murder."

Framing the Issue as Killing

The issue of helping a patient die is confusing because it is inevitably confused with euthanasia, or "mercy killing." As we have noted, euthanasia is intentionally ending someone else's life in the belief that the person's death would be a kinder mercy than prolonging his or her life. But it becomes a slippery slope when it shifts from ending the life of someone who is dying to ending the life of someone whose life others judge to be substandard. It is for this reason that the disabled have been in the forefront of resisting physician-assisted death. Some fear PAD could rapidly devolve into euthanasia—and such a policy would raise the inevitable question, Whose life is considered worth living and whose is not? The human rights concerns such a question raises are clearly legitimate. But what might we learn about our humanity by considering how we approach the topic of euthanasia?

In our society, we routinely euthanize dying animals to prevent their suffering. In fact, in many cases we euthanize animals that are *not* dying, such as racehorses that have sustained career-ending fractures or stray cats or dogs that remain unclaimed. Why, we may ask, are we willing to prevent the suffering of dying animals through euthanasia while not willing to do the same for our own species? What exactly is the difference?

For one thing, we have no means of asking animals if it is what they want. Thus we take it upon ourselves to make the decision for them—and do not presume, as was done in the case of Terri Schiavo or Nancy Cruzan, that they could ever make the decision. We choose "mercy killing" or euthanasia for suffering animals because we are compassionate and don't want them to suffer. We assume it is in their best interest—but how do we really know? The truth is, we don't. But we do have enough information to make reasonable judgments weighing the value of a dying animal's life against its suffering.

If making these decisions is allowable for animals, how do we justify *not* doing the same for humans? Why doesn't the same reasoning and compassion apply to our own species? Because for one thing, according to scripture, the sanctity of life applies only to humans, not animals.

Leon Kass, a physician, scientist, and educator, was the chairman of George W. Bush's President's Council on Bioethics from 2001 to 2005. In an article he wrote in 1991, opposing a "right to die" initiative, he rhetorically asked the question of why, if we put animals out of their misery, is it not inhumane to allow the same for humans.[23] To his question he answered:

Perhaps inhumane, but not thereby inhuman. On the contrary, it is precisely because animals are not human that we must treat them (merely) humanely. We put dumb animals to sleep because they do not know that they are dying, because they can make nothing of their misery or mortality, and, therefore, because they cannot live deliberately—i.e., humanly—in the face of their own suffering and dying. They cannot live out a fitting end. ... Humanity is owed humanity, not humaneness.[24]

There you have it—we are allowed to treat animals humanely, but we should not treat humans "humanely" but "humanly." Kass does not mention the scriptural basis for his explanation but rather distinguishes between human and humane with a semantic gyration. What a difference one letter makes in a word! True, most people don't respect the lives of animals (think chickens, cows, lambs, or pigs), and it seems highly unlikely that animals can conceptualize "God's will" as we do. But couldn't animals have an understanding of their state of health, or mortality, in a nonhuman manner? Moreover, what is to be made of Kass's claim that "animals do not know they are dying"? Such a statement flies in the face of zoology and biology, where the death rituals of animals are as much a source of fascination and speculation as are birth or mating rituals. And it hardly takes a visit to the Discovery channel to grasp the intuitions of the animal kingdom that death is near. As any pet owner knows, cats and dogs will wander off to die, finding a secluded spot hidden from human view and access, such as going to the woods, or hiding in the back of a closet. Why would they do that if they didn't have an awareness that they are dying?

The answer is in a particular belief and understanding of God, in which, of course, animals presumably don't participate. But that's exactly the point, according to sanctity-of-life orthodoxy. Humans alone among the animals are considered able to understand and commune with God. The semantic gyration over human and humane is an attempt to offset a glaring contradiction in the "God's will" argument (discussed in more detail in chapter 3). It is a cover for an authoritative set of beliefs that are presumed to be true and which explain a range of social beliefs and behaviors. How, then, have these beliefs come to be applied to the concept of assisted death?

The answer once again can be found in the art of framing—in this case, framing assisted death as an act of killing.

Assisted Dying as Killing

"The role of the physician is to affirm human life, relieve suffering, and give compassionate, competent care as long as the patient lives. The physician as well as the patient will be held accountable by God, the giver and taker of life."[25]

The belief in divine control over life and death is the springboard of the Judeo-Christian tradition. This belief is incorporated in the powerful principle of "the sanctity of life," specifically of *human* life. Under this paradigm, inherited from the Jewish tradition and expanded under Christianity, since every human is formed in the image of God, and it is God who gives life, life is therefore holy or sanctified. Thus, abortion, euthanasia, and suicide are viewed as sins against God's work, and under the principle of the sanctity of life, physicians were and still are enjoined from helping their patients die, regardless of circumstances. And this principle is the foundation of opposition to physician aid in dying for most who oppose the practice.

Although some who oppose physician aid in dying do so for professional, legal, or secular ethical concerns, the most forceful, protracted opposition to PAD is based on the religious precept of the act being a form of killing and thus a sin against God's will—which therefore merits punishment. To disapprove of PAD for this reason is, therefore, unquestionably a legitimate "free exercise of religion" as granted by the First Amendment to the

US Constitution. Nevertheless, it is important to understand how this precept operates in our society, and how the "free exercise of religion" can effectively serve to ban or prevent others from access to certain medical procedures that their own religion may not prohibit—or in some cases, from the exercise of their own religious views. After all, to the person who feels that using technology to maintain a persistent vegetative state when natural death would occur without it, thus preventing the release of their soul, the denial of death may be viewed as a sin against God's will. How, then, does society reconcile these conflicting views?

Thou shalt not kill.—Exodus 20:13, KJV, translated from Hebrew

Is physician-assisted dying contrary to the sanctity of life? Does intervention with the intent to produce death for the relief of suffering violate the sanctity of life? The oldest Judeo-Christian injunction against taking the life of another human being comes from the Ten Commandments as given by God to Moses. If we are to accept that the commandment "Thou shalt not kill," which is listed in two books of the Hebrew Bible: Exodus 20:1–17 and Deuteronomy 5:4–21, and listed variously as the fifth or sixth commandment[26] is actually the word of God, we are still left begging the question: What does it mean "to kill"?

Lexicographers define "to kill" as "to deprive of life," but without condition. "Kill" merely states the fact. Thus, one is killed by a falling tree, or by a heart attack, or by a bullet. "To deprive of life" implies an act, or omission of a life-saving act, but makes no judgment whether the "killing" of another person is intended, desired or undesired, or accepted by the community. Nor does it take into account the viability of the person who dies. By strict definition, the word does not imply a wrongful act; it says only, "but for the act, the person would not have died." Nevertheless, the word "kill" commonly carries the connotation of illegality, wickedness, or sinfulness.

Of course, the injunction "Thou shalt not kill," as well as respect for life, are the bedrock of all ethical systems, although killing in some forms is sanctioned in all societies. We generally accept that we may kill nonhuman life forms, such as those we define as pests or predators or disease pathogens. While "mercy killing" of suffering humans is widely condemned, few condemn the mercy killing of suffering animals. All human societies have advocated hunting animals as a means to survival, although cultures and people within cultures vary on whether it is acceptable to hunt animals for sport. Societies also provide exceptions to the killing of people. We almost always agree that it is acceptable to kill people in self-defense. Some societies sanction the killing of criminals; curiously, those who most vociferously condemn assisted death on the grounds that it is a violation of Christian ethics are sometimes the most vociferous advocates of capital punishment for certain crimes.

But indisputably, war is the greatest sanctioned form of killing, and it is one that almost all human societies have engaged in and condone in one form or another. Nonetheless, even in the context of war, rules remain which help regulate when and how killing is to be carried out. Within the Christian tradition, St. Augustine framed the concept of a just war, and centuries later, Thomas Aquinas used the authority of Augustine's arguments in an attempt to define the conditions under which a war could be just in order to save other lives, to defend just societies, or to achieve peace.[27] Also, according to Augustine, God may command a killing, as he did when he commanded Isaac be sacrificed.[28]

Clearly, the lives of soldiers killed in combat and civilians killed by "collateral damage" are rationalized by society as acceptable killing because the loss of these lives is viewed as necessary for "just" purposes. But as history teaches us, all wars, regardless of who carries them out and for what aim, and regardless of whether there was any provocation, are always launched in the name of self-defense. Even Hitler persuaded his followers that his mission was in defense of the German nation. The moral prohibition against killing is circumvented in this way by justifying warfare as defensive—in other words, killing can be made acceptable if it is believed to be done to *prevent* other people from being killed.

Moreover, justification of killing "to defend just societies" presumes "justness" of the society doing the killing and "unjustness" of the society of the people who are killed, a presumption mostly false over the ages—but necessary to legitimate warfare.

In addition, because humans have an aversion to killing other humans, when a nation and its people go to war, those who are deemed "the enemy" will be referred to in dehumanizing terms, such as "terrorists," "evildoers," "commies," "reds," "gooks," or "vermin."[29] By using dehumanizing terms to reference those who are to be killed, they are viewed as less than human, their killing made all the more acceptable.

The long history and global spread of warfare has demonstrated that as long as warfare can be convincingly represented as a necessary act, and a form of justice through the principle of self-defense or a "just war," it will be widely accepted and serve to unite a population against its perceived enemy. So strong is this view that societies will turn with a united vengeance against their own citizens who do not join in the collective call for bloodshed, as we have seen whenever war protestors speak out against our nation's wars.

Over the last two millennia, thousands, or hundreds of thousands of "heretics" were beheaded or burned at the stake in the name of defending presumed "just" institutions and peoples. Indeed, mass killing proffered by the Crusades was not just acceptable but incited under the rubric of defending a just society—that is, the Church—while trying to destroy an "evil" society. These same social processes continue throughout the world to this day as nations and their citizens—including deeply religious ones—send their youth to kill and be killed over territory, resources, principles, and identities, giving pause to any argument that assisted death for the suffering is a violation of the sanctity of life.

Thus, all societies allow some types of killing while prohibiting others. In our own society, whose life is sanctified? And how is the sanctity of life violated? Because society does not disallow killing per se, we must understand how the institutions of government and religion make the necessarily arbitrary distinctions between allowable and nonallowable killing. They make these distinctions through framing.

Murder or Killing? It's All in a Word

You shall not murder.—Exodus 20:13, NKJV, NIV, and ESV

The major objection to physician-assisted dying thus rests on a narrow, human-derived interpretation that human life is holy, or must be *sanctified*, as determined for the most part by institutional ideology. The word "kill," as most people use it, is too simplistic and inadequate to the task of defining physicians' practices in a fair, uniform, and enlightened manner by which we may advance our understanding of what physicians' clinical practices entail. However, language is crucial to shaping attitudes about end-of-life practices. The words one uses to define a procedure may carry a formative value judgment. The use or avoidance of "kill" seems intended more to shape attitudes than to describe specific acts. If we are to use the word "kill" in describing practices, we must apply a uniform definition in assessing various other end-of-life medical practices, some of which actually fulfill the definition of killing but are not called such. When *kill* is used by those who oppose PAD, it is another example of reliance on the religious principle of sanctity of life.

According to modern versions of the Bible, it is *murder*, not killing, that is prohibited. And murder, according to the Bible and secular definitions, is the unlawful taking of a human life. In legal terms, murder is the unlawful killing of a human being by another human being, with malicious aforethought (while manslaughter is the unlawful killing of a human through negligence or reckless indifference to the consequences of one's actions or nonactions).

So does physician-assisted dying constitute murder, as Heracles's son—and, as we will see, many modern physicians—so feared? Is there "malice aforethought"? Certainly there is intent to help the patient die, but when it is done to *help* the patient, to comply with the patient's desire and request, it is a form of helping, with no malice inherent. Is it thus wrongful murder? Maybe it is to others who object to it ideologically, but not to the person asking for it.

But the most important reason physician-assisted dying is not murder is that it lacks the legal requirement of "an unlawful *killing of a human being by another human being.*" This may be what happens with involuntary euthanasia, but it does not happen in PAD as I propose the concept. Through PAD, the patient, not the physician, commits the act of ending his or her life—there is no killing of one person by another. And while some may argue that because the physician provides assistance in the form of the lethal agent, it is tantamount to killing, I would counter that the same logic could be applied to gun sales—yet the gun dealer who is providing lethal weapons is doing so with far less concern for the consequences of this assistance. But unlike Jack Kevorkian, who was ultimately imprisoned not for his self-described "suicide machine" but for injecting the lethal medicines, PAD as proposed here is a form of assistance to the patient by providing a resource. Neither the physician nor the gun merchant kills the patient by providing him or her the means to do so. Yet by framing the issue of assisted death as a "sanctity of life issue," it has become embraced as a "right-to-life" and, hence, conservative political issue.

Thus, as many of those who oppose physician-assisted dying advocate for another cause near and dear to the conservative heart—unrestricted gun rights—they forcefully advocate for the rights of gun dealers to sell not only handguns but assault rifles, machine guns, and even grenade launchers, and to not be held accountable for what their customers do with these weapons once they have them. The response to gun control that has been summarily dismissed with the slogan, "Guns don't kill people, people kill people" could just as logically be applied to PAD. "Pills don't kill people, people kill themselves." Why then is this argument distinguishing the actor from the lethal object applied to one set of beliefs but not the other?

Such seemingly disparate social positions—the right to own and sell military assault rifles against the denial of the right to provide or obtain medicines to help the dying die more painlessly— has been presented as a unified belief system, reflecting logically and morally consistent positions rather than the contradictory positions they clearly are. And in so doing, while the issue of gun rights is framed as an inalienable constitutional right that protects the citizen from control of the government, the issue of physician-assisted death has been presented as something meriting greater control from the government. This logic suggests that our society needs fewer laws controlling lethal weapons but greater laws controlling how we die.

How has this contrary logic been packaged and sold to the American public? By framing it with the religious principles of the sanctity of human life and the right to life. But whose rights, and whose lives, merit protection are a matter of social standing. The "unborn" are considered by those who embrace a right-to-life viewpoint as having lives meriting protection and government mandate. Yet once they are born, if they have any health problems, these same right-to-life advocates are likely to have a different view, arguing that extending resources that could save lives is not considered a right in the United States unless the child's parents can afford insurance. It is remarkable that a child can be born into this country and throughout life be deprived of rights to health care because they don't have insurance, yet if their lack of health care leads to their early death, our state will find the means to prolong their suffering by investing in long-term care that keeps them alive in a vegetative state! Any arguments for "sanctity of life" or "right-to-life" are specious, in my view, because these are not so credible as they are convenient, being invoked to disregard life just as readily as they are invoked to protect life. How else to explain why those who block any efforts that might make assisted dying legal almost always support and celebrate capital punishment and warfare, deny access to life-saving health care to those who can't afford it, and vigorously defend those who manufacture, sell, and stockpile AK-47s? Well, there is one way to explain it. And that is to hide the right-to-life argument under the rug altogether when that argument just won't cut it.

The Great Deception—Undercover Ideology

With the highly politicized death of Terri Schiavo, opponents framed the issue of PAD as one of right to life. In so doing, they shifted the argument from one of patients' rights to one of civil rights. As all politicians know, if the other side wants to talk about a certain subject, so long as you talk about why that subject is not important and should not be the issue, the listener will be hard-pressed to think of anything but that subject.

Similarly, by describing assisted death as a right-to-life issue—a term long used for the highly politicized topic of abortion—any argument in support of assisted death or even natural death through the removal of life support becomes characterized as a denial of someone's "right" to life. The right-to-death argument consequently remained off the table once those who opposed that right seized the linguistic high ground and moved the discourse from one of sanctity of life (where the concept of "mercy killing" resides) to one of a right to life (where the concept of "killing" resides). And in a nation based on inalienable rights, once PAD was framed as a rights issue, opponents had found their platform. Yet there was still a troubling obstacle—not everyone shared their views. For all the visibility the politicized right-to-life movement has gained in recent years, it remains a minority view in our nation. Thus, to defeat laws that could ensure the right to PAD, it sometimes becomes necessary to obscure the underlying religious ideology of the opposition while simultaneously strengthening it.

This duplicitous approach struck me recently while watching a recent televised spat over whether all women should have a vaginal ultrasound test prior to abortion. A woman from one of the right-to-life organizations said, "This is a medical issue—it's a matter of informed consent." She went on to argue that a vaginal ultrasound was necessary for a woman to give consent for an abortion, and that doing so was a matter of "best medical practice." To the counterargument that passing a law to force women to have this invasive test was a violation of privacy and was mandating a medical practice, the woman stuck to her theme of "it's necessary to provide optimal medical care—it's strictly a health-care issue." Yet, is it? After all, many who oppose abortion believe that even if an abortion is necessary to protect or even save the life of the mother, it should still be denied, and a primary goal of the National Right to Life Coalition is to shut down access to health care provided by Planned Parenthood and other clinics. Treating abortion as a health-care issue is rarely if ever a concern of opponents when actual health-care issues are raised.

One of the goals of framing is to present the issue so there is only one possible answer, thereby excluding other answers. In the five- or six-minute debate on the issue, after the speaker was introduced as a member of a "right-to-life" organization, the role of religion underpinning the right-to-life goal of preventing abortions was never even mentioned. The framing of a religious belief as a "health-care issue" was successful in keeping the debate focused entirely on what constitutes good medical practice and not whether every woman should have medical care as directed by a certain ideology. Controlling the discussion is key.

In debates surrounding attempts to pass laws allowing physician aid in dying, opponents similarly keep their ideology undercover and argue on strictly secular grounds. The major opponents are usually—almost always—individuals with strong ties to fundamentalist religious groups. For example, when I was involved in passage of Initiative-1000, the Washington state "death-with-dignity" statute allowing physician aid in dying, during public debates I noted that with few exceptions the physician speakers who denounced the bill belonged to the Christian Medical Association (CMA), an organization that strongly opposes physician aid in dying on religious grounds. Nevertheless, even including a Catholic deacon, none of the speakers I heard during the campaign used religion to support their opposition to physician aid in dying, or in any way referred to their religious beliefs, even though their positions on PAD were directly related to their religious beliefs.

Thus, in a curious but understandable political strategy, opponents of physician aid in dying have taken their ideology underground. It seems it isn't always politically helpful for them to tout their version of God's will in political disputes. Americans on the whole may be quite religious, but not many voters are pleased to have a religious group lecture them on morality or tell them how they should vote in an election. It's one thing to hear the clergy of one's own group give the party line of the faithful, but it's quite another matter to have someone else's representative touting their religion and telling you how to vote. Consequently, religious groups have learned to keep a low profile on their ideology while resorting to civil—or secular—arguments and methods in political campaigns.

Another example from Washington state's right-to-die initiative that I was involved with in 1991 involved an intelligent, well-spoken nun who was the director of the Washington State Catholic Conference, which represents the Catholic bishops on issues of public policy. As the leading speaker of the opposition to the bill, she used only secular arguments to promote her position, which helped make her an effective spokesperson for the opposition to the initiative, which subsequently failed to pass.

But by 2008, when the Death with Dignity Act was once again put to a vote, the social tides had changed. In the buildup before the official start of the campaign for the law, proponents emphasized her religious affiliation and beliefs, from which she could not hide in her nun's habit. In my opinion, although she was a more capable speaker than most of the others the opponents had to offer, because her ideological orientation had been unmasked, she rarely—if at all—spoke publicly during the actual political campaign. Instead, in order to avoid the strong ideological connection to opposition to physician aid in dying, opponents primarily used physicians who shared the opposition ideology but spoke in strictly medical or secular terms. Because the social tides had turned and were no longer on their side, it became a political necessity for the opposition to go underground with their underlying ideology supporting their opposition and use a more secular approach. But their efforts failed, and in 2008 Washington's Death with Dignity Act was made into law.

Opponents to PAD have recognized that religious arguments are not as effective in uniting the multitudes as they might hope. Consequently, their standard mode of public operation has now become to use *only* secular arguments and to avoid sectarian religious references altogether. Even someone as staunchly religious as Wesley Smith, a senior fellow at the Discovery Institute, which is the driving force behind efforts to stop educators from teaching evolution in favor of teaching "intelligent design" and "affirming the reality of God,"[30] has found the secular approach effective. In addition to his goals of ridding the world of evolutionary theory, Smith has testified in opposition to the legalization of physician-assisted suicide before the California Senate Judiciary Committee, stating, "My work in the fields in which I advocate is entirely secular."[31] And in keeping with the strategy of avoiding ideological arguments, what he said was entirely secular, as he made no mention of the religiously conservative, right-to-life ideology underlying his and the Discovery Institute's work.

Unlike their forebears of two millennia ago, ideological opponents of physician aid in dying hide their true colors—and in so doing, perpetrate a great deception on the public.

Taking Care to Hide Ideology

The religious efforts to undermine physician-assisted death have gone one step further, to take aim even at advance directives. An advance directive, or "living will," is a document signed by a patient that clearly states his or her wishes regarding health care in the event the person is incapacitated and unable to make decisions. Advance directives typically name someone to have decision-making authority over the patient's care and include instructions pertaining to what he or she desires concerning life support, resuscitation orders, and pain relief.

In 2005, under the chairmanship of Leon Kass, the President's Council on Bioethics published *Taking Care*, an outline of a conservative agenda on medical ethics.[32] Throughout this 223-page report the authors denigrate autonomy in medical decision making as being selfish and often in conflict with others' moral concepts. The authors conclude that advance directives should be opposed because "no individual can foresee every future circumstance; and medical situations are so complex that we can only judge wisely what to do case-by-case and in the moment."

In advocating against advance directives, President Bush's Council on Bioethics attempted to disregard decades of consensus in medical ethics that patients have the right to self-determine their medical courses based on their individual values and goals. Instead, the council urged caregivers to replace end-of-life medical decision making with a uniform approach to all patients. To do this, they resorted to the concept of "equality" as the highest principle of medical ethics, by which they said all patients should be treated equally. But by this they meant by applying *their* moral standard to everyone and not allowing anyone the right to PAD in any form—not even to have an advance directive honored.

According to the logic advanced in *Taking Care*, "Our caregivers are not obligated to execute our wishes if those wishes seem morally misguided, nor obligated to enter into contracts that require them to violate important moral precepts that are binding on everyone."[33] In other words, disregard the patients' wishes if you disagree with them, just so long as your disagreements are in accordance with the values of the right-to-life faction.

Another position made in *Taking Care* used to justify disregarding advance directives is the claim that physicians are concerned with the "here and now" rather than a patient's past wishes. While on the surface such an argument might be interpreted as justifying keeping a patient alive only if new and unforeseen medical breakthroughs have made a once irreversible medical condition a recoverable one, that is not the way they intend their position to be applied. If it were, advance directives would not be so uniformly rejected by the council. The argument that the patient be kept alive regardless of his or her medical condition and *stated wishes* is yet another example of religious ideology being masked as a scientific concern. Moreover, it isn't even sensible. If one applied this "here-and-now" principle to ordinary wills, executors of a deceased person could disregard a person's will and allocate the estate according to their version of what is morally best.

Needless to say, the moral precept the president's council wanted to impose on us all is *their* conception of what is moral, which in turn is deeply ideological and based on the sanctity-of-life principle but dressed as "equality." As Dr. Janet Rowley, a dissenting member of the President's Council on Bioethics, wrote regarding the recommendation that advanced directives may be overridden, "this report is scary."[34]

The Consequences of Ideological Control over Public Issues

In the debate over physician aid in dying, the positions of various medical associations matter a lot, as they are taken to reflect the collective thinking and recommendations of physicians who are, after all, the ones who should best know what is good or bad for their patients. There are hundreds of medical societies or organizations on the national, state, county, and even city levels, but the best known to the general public are the American Medical Association

(AMA) and the state medical associations that are branches of the AMA. Although other national medical organizations such as the American Cancer Society and the American Heart Association are very important and exercise considerable political weight on issues pertaining to their membership, the AMA and its state affiliates are politically most visible and generally exercise the most clout with national and state legislatures, as well as with state voter initiatives.

In steadfastly opposing any effort to make physician aid in dying legal, however, the AMA and its state affiliates have misrepresented the broader medical community as well as their narrower base of members. For example, Initiative-1000, the 2008 state of Washington ballot issue I was involved in, displayed the political power and workings of an ideologically opposed minority. Since at least 1991, the Washington State Medical Association (WSMA) had opposed, in a resolution approved by its House of Delegates, any form of physician aid in dying. Resolutions passed by delegates are the mechanism for policy-making for most medical associations.

Two years before Initiative-1000, in 2006, I and another proponent of physician aid in dying submitted to the WSMA a resolution for "neutrality" on the issue, to supersede the old resolution against physician aid in dying. We took this action in anticipation of Initiative-1000 being on the ballot in a year or two. Our resolution for neutrality had already gained approval of the King County (Seattle) Medical Society. We did not ask the WSMA for approval of or support for physician aid in dying—just neutrality. Obviously, the recommendation of the largest medical group in the state would be very important in any election on the issue, and we thought this approach was fair since we would not be asking the WSMA to support a procedure some of its members opposed on ideological grounds.

Here's the way this process works. When the WSMA holds its annual meeting, there may be thirty to fifty resolutions submitted from around the state for consideration. Each resolution is assigned to one of several "reference" committees, each headed by a chair and assistant chair. Each reference committee has hearings on all the resolutions assigned to it, with the goal of allowing every individual who wishes to speak on the subject the opportunity to do so. At the end of the hearing, the chair and assistant chair make a recommendation to approve or disapprove the resolution, presumably based on consideration of the evidence and the views expressed by the representative speakers.

When our resolution came up for discussion, the other cosponsor introduced it briefly, and then I spoke for about a minute in favor of it. When I was through I noticed about fifteen people already in line to speak, more than the usual total for a resolution. One by one these physicians then took the microphone to oppose the resolution, each attacking our proposition from a different angle, only to be echoed by another procession of at least ten more speakers. Some evoked God's purpose, many evoked Hippocrates, and virtually all called PAD killing, and, in two instances, murder. The protests took about forty-five minutes, and during that time only one other speaker supported the resolution, but only in the most modest terms. Needless to say, the sense of the meeting was totally against us, so my colleague and I withdrew our resolution.

When the session was over, a friend who had for many years opposed physician-assisted dying but was now neutral on the issue asked me what I thought about the hearing.

"Wow," I said, "that sounded orchestrated."

"Well, it was," he answered. "Didn't you know that?"

"No, how would I have known that?"

"Oh, they networked with everyone they knew who was against physician aid in dying to get them to attend the annual meeting and speak against your resolution."

I was astounded. In point of fact, he told me, a representative of the Washington State Catholic Conference had contacted him and every physician who had lined up against physician aid in dying during a prior initiative in 1991, plus more added to the list since then. Their mobilization was overwhelming. Anyone present at that hearing would have concluded that more than 90 percent of Washington state physicians were against the resolution when, in fact, they represented a minority viewpoint. But they were effective at organizing themselves, and their strategic mobilization succeeded at presenting an image of consensus, when no such consensus existed.

Yes, I was politically naïve, but with encouragement from like-minded colleagues I tried a similar resolution the following year, again asking for neutrality on the issue. But this time I did my own networking; I spoke to many individual physicians and to medical groups, explaining how we got ambushed the year before, and asking for their participation in support of another resolution. Well, dear reader, you know what happened—exactly the same thing. The opposition still managed to do a better job at making their voices heard.

I never learned who had managed the opponents' networking the second time, or how they managed to do it so well, but it was extremely effective. Some physicians speaking against the resolution shed tears as they spoke of their fear of this ungodly proposal. And as for the physicians I had lined up? In contrast to the approximately thirty-five speakers against, there were only three who would willingly speak in support of the resolution. While those who opposed it did not fear their views were unpopular, in contrast, those who supported it were fearful of speaking out.

The resolution was doomed, and I learned from some insiders that when supporters learned how many physicians were lined up to speak against it if it got to the full assembly, they backed down. In light of their resistance, we withdrew the resolution and accepted that we would not get the endorsement of our state's medical association no matter how many members privately supported it.

The way these resolutions were defeated was a remarkable example of the mobilizing power of ideology. On one hand, those with strong ideologies in opposition to PAD responded willingly and vigorously; they had no inhibitions in stating their values and goals and protecting the institutions they represented. On the other hand, of the many who supported physician aid in dying, very few were willing to "stick their necks out" on a controversial subject. They didn't (and don't) want to be in conflict with other medical colleagues, friends, or patients. The reason they back down so readily when their counterparts do not is because they have no ideology to protect. As the wife of one delegate to both WSMA conventions told me, "My husband is a physician, not an activist." And that is the problem in a nutshell—the opposition may be a minority, but they are an activist minority. Protesters gather outside of offices of physicians who perform abortions, not at the offices of doctors who oppose it. That is the way ideology works. It unites people in opposition to a perceived enemy and the public responds to the fear any enemy presents.

As disheartening as this experience was, the story has a more regrettable, even ominous aspect. As I said above, the AMA and its affiliate WSMA have misrepresented and do misrepresent physicians on this issue. As a starter, fewer than half of the physicians in Washington state belong to the WSMA, and those who do belong tend to be more politically conservative than nonmembers. And because the organization is comprised of so many conservative members, those who are not conservative are less likely to join, only reinforcing the strength and political influence of its conservative membership. By this measure alone, the WSMA cannot claim to speak for the physicians of the state. Even more telling, however, is a survey of members that the WSMA commissioned in 2007. The survey covered many subjects, was done by a respected pollster, and was representative of the WSMA membership.

One question asked:

> Would you support a ballot measure that makes physician-assisted suicide legal and defines physician-assisted suicide as a practice in which the physician provides a terminally ill patient with a lethal dose

of medication, upon the patient's request, which the patient intends to use to end his or her life?[35]

The result was that 50 percent said they would support such a measure, and 42 percent would oppose it. Thus, half of all WSMA members actually supported a ballot measure exactly like the pro-assisted dying Initiative-1000!

Yet even though the WSMA had this information in hand as early as March 2007, they chose not to release it. Worse, they went on public record as opposing physician aid in dying, and in 2008 opposed Initiative-1000. Prior to the election the results of the survey were ultimately made public by the *Seattle Times*.[36]

After learning of this survey, I asked some of the WSMA leaders and others who had spoken against the resolution why they had refused to release the survey to the public and why they didn't take it as reason for the medical association to at least not openly oppose the initiative. The answer was uniformly that "the study was no good and no one should believe it." But the survey was actually very well designed, scientific and accurate. And incredibly, even after the survey was made public, physicians opposed to I-1000 kept telling public audiences, "Washington state physicians are *against* this initiative." So much for these physicians' notion of "evidence-based medicine." Despite their scientific training, it seems that just like anybody else, when physicians don't like the evidence, they merely ignore it.

Despite the opposition of the WSMA, the voters of Washington did pass the initiative for PAD in 2008. Nevertheless, in 2011 the opposition made an attempt to eviscerate it through political pressure, when the WSMA lobbied the legislature to require physicians to state the cause of death as "suicide" on the death certificates of patients who died under the law. Because it is relatively easy to access death certificates, opponents could then identify physicians acting under the law and expose them in the same way they expose physicians who perform abortions. If that were to happen, physicians would be much more reluctant to use the law. At best, this was nasty politics aimed to thwart the will of the public. At worst, it was a classic example of how a minority sought to interfere with patients' legal rights to health care by distorting, fabricating, and lying about evidence supporting that legal right. Any way you cut it, the move was ugly.

Fortunately, we were able to advise the WSMA delegates about the purpose of this underhanded move, and the resolution to alter the law was defeated.

So, given this experience, what should we expect on the national level? Sadly, the same thing. The AMA claims to speak for doctors, and the media often echo that assertion, yet barely a quarter of the nation's physicians are members of the AMA. Nevertheless, as noted above, the AMA has long opposed physician aid in dying, as "incompatible with the physician's role of healing."[37] While this remains the official position of the AMA, and was crafted by 430 physicians in the AMA House of Delegates, it never accurately reflected its membership. Independent investigators released a nationwide survey of AMA members in 2001 regarding attitudes toward legalization of physician aid in dying and the results indicated that only one-third actually opposed it. While fewer than half (44.5 percent) favored legalization, nearly a quarter (22 percent) were unsure.[38]

But the reason the AMA has been so successful at representing the issue as if a majority did in fact oppose PAD is because its leadership strongly opposes it. Whereas a plurality of the general membership of the AMA supported legal physician aid in dying as cited above, among members of the AMA House of Delegates, which shapes policy, 61.6 percent opposed legalization, 23.5 percent favored legalization, and 15 percent were unsure. That is, the policy-directing House of Delegates held views on the subject that essentially represented just the opposite of what the general membership believes. The AMA, just like the WSMA, thus provides us with yet another example of how a minority group can politically control a large medical institution on a matter of ideology. These examples show the organizing power of ideology in working to advance their views in opposition to the majority.

Framing the Issue as Suicide

We have thus far seen how the issue of assisted death has been opposed by framing it as a civil rights issue, a health-care issue, and a right-to-life issue. But what to make of the patient who rejects such a "right" to life and begs to die? Well, that becomes framed as a case of suicide—and as such, a mental-health issue. For no one in a rational state of mind would end his or her own life, according to this framework. But what happens when someone, such as the fictional Ken Harrison or the very real David Rivlin, proves his or her sanity and still asks for help with dying? Well then, that must be the work of the devil. According to Thomas Aquinas, "life is a gift made to man by God, and it is subject to him who is master of death and life. Therefore, a person who takes his own life sins against God."[39]

Arguably, the Christian doctrine of everlasting life as reward for good deeds has prompted suicides, for much the same reason as occurs now with Islamists who accept suicide missions against perceived enemies of their faith. But from the fourth century, when Augustine determined that suicide constituted a form of killing, it has been viewed among many Christians as a sin for which there is no repentance. Augustine based this conclusion on the commandment "Thou shalt not kill," extending it to include oneself as well as others who must not be killed.[40] To Augustine, the only form of killing allowed, of self or others, is killing carried out at the orders of divine authority, which is to say, by God.[41]

In later years, St. Thomas Aquinas also defended this prohibition, saying suicide violates our duty to God because God has given us life as a gift, and in taking our lives we violate his right to determine the duration of our earthly existence.[42] This conclusion was codified in the medieval doctrine that suicide nullified human beings' relationship with God, under the belief that our control over our body is limited to rights of possession, while God retains dominion over that possession.[43]

Whatever may be the doctrinal prohibitions against suicide, we must examine whether PAD is suicide in the linguistic sense of the word. Just as we have seen how important it is to examine the meaning of the word "kill," we must also ask, "What is the perceived meaning of the word suicide?" Although the most common interpretation is of a violent, secretive, sinful act, we have seen the word includes other forms of socially or culturally acceptable self-dying, and so has a spectrum of meanings, ranging from vile to laudable. In other words, although the word *suicide* presents as "one size fits all,"—like the word "kill,"—it is not sufficient to cover a broad range of different meanings.

The problem is a linguistic deficiency. Margaret Pabst Battin, a philosopher of medical ethics, shows the limitations of a single word for the various forms of "self-caused death" by comparing the English word *suicide* with several German words, all meaning "self-caused death" but carrying different connotations.[44] Whereas the word *selbstmord*, the most-used German term for self-inflicted death, carries extremely negative connotations, the word *freitod* means "free death" or "voluntary death," and is associated with individual choice and therefore not associated with moral wrongness. In contrast, the single English word *suicide* does not distinguish among differing types of self-caused death. As a result, it limits our ability to conceptualize it and smears the practice of PAD with the connotation of a repugnant or sinful act. This deficiency applies not just to PAD but even to Catholic Church doctrines. While the Church condemns PAD as suicide, it simultaneously teaches that, "One must clearly distinguish suicide from that sacrifice of one's life whereby for a higher cause, such as God's glory, the salvation of souls or the service of one's brethren, a person offers his or her own life or puts it in danger."[45] Clearly, context matters. Whether one uses the term suicide to describe an act of self-caused death depends not only on the act itself but on one's ideological beliefs.

Just as Samson in the Bible accepted his own death when he toppled the pillars of the Philistines' temple, praying to God as he did so, "Let me die with the Philistines!" (Judges 16:30, KJV), the passengers who brought down the hijacked airliner in Pennsylvania on 9/11 were hailed as heroes, not as suicides. When they brought the plane down, they caused their own deaths and those of everyone on board. But they did so not to end their lives but to avert an even greater tragedy even though they knew they would die in the process. Because of the circumstances in which they gave their lives, we don't say they "committed suicide." We say they were honorable and valiant by giving their lives the way they did. They knew they were going to die regardless, so they chose the best way to die. Physician aid in dying is the same—the patient is going to die and chooses the least dreadful way of going.

Nonetheless, the stigma of suicide has long colored discussions of PAD, and with it, enabled religious ideology to frame social policies pertaining to PAD as a violation of God's will. This use of religion to justify social policies has a long and troubled history.

The eighteenth-century philosopher David Hume was concerned with the manner in which religion was used to invoke a range of social policies under the guise of divine authority. Among his arguments was that prohibiting suicide as a violation of God's will was nonsensical. To save the life of someone otherwise dying, he reasoned, was equally intervening with God's will, but not one any rational person would suggest not be done. In an essay on suicide that he instructed not be published until after his death, no doubt owing to the heated sentiment the topic provoked, Hume wrote, "That suicide may often be consistent with interest and with our duty to *ourselves* no one can question, who allows that age, sickness, or misfortune may render life a burden, and make it worse than annihilation."[46]

Writing nearly a century later, the German philosopher Schopenhauer was also confident about the rationality of suicide: "It will generally be found that, as soon as the terrors of life outweigh the terrors of death, a man will put an end to his life."[47]

Yet the AMA—the premier medical association in the United States—both rejects these views and sides with the religious right as it promotes the framing of PAD as an act of suicide: "allowing physicians to participate in assisted suicide would cause more harm than good. Physician-assisted suicide is fundamentally incompatible with the physician's role as healer, would be difficult or impossible to control, and would pose serious societal risks."[48]

But is the commonly held meaning of "suicide" an appropriate conceptual framework for physician-assisted dying? When we explore the meanings of suicide, we find it is not. When PAD became widely discussed in the 1990s and beyond, it was almost uniformly called physician-assisted suicide. Unfortunately, this terminology gave supporters of PAD a semantic difficulty. From a strictly etymological angle, physician aid in dying *is* suicide, as the root *sui* means "self," and *cide* means "death." But that's where the accuracy ends, when the word is used to describe physician aid in dying. Framing PAD as suicide is not only misleading, it is inaccurate.

There are several major differences between physician aid in dying and suicide. First, PAD is only for a patient who has an irreversible and incurable *terminal* disease. As I and most advocates of PAD in the United States firmly believe, assisting the death of anyone who is not terminally ill should not be legal. In contrast, true, or ordinary suicide, is the self-inflicted death of someone who is suffering from an illness (whether emotional or physical) that is in almost all cases treatable, if not curable, *and they would not die in the foreseeable future were it not for the act of suicide.*[49] In this view, the majority of the actions of Jack Kevorkian, for example, could rightly be termed "assisted suicide" because many of the people he helped to die were suffering from treatable conditions such as arthritis, diabetes, or back pain, or from psychosomatic illnesses with no evidence of anything physically wrong with them. (When he directly injected the lethal drug into some of his patients, however, it was euthanasia, not assisted suicide.)

Second, and importantly, a suicide is almost always secretive, done without notification to family and friends, and it is often violent, as with a gun, slashing an artery open, hanging, or jumping from a bridge. Suicide causes great shock and despair for families, and the resulting psychological harm to loved ones, friends, and colleagues is great, lasting, and often devastating. It is the ultimate antisocial act of departure, a rupture of the community of the individual with others, and leaves those left behind angry, confused, and remorseful for the rest of their lives.

Physician-assisted dying or aid in dying is quite the opposite. In addition to being a peaceful death, it gives patients and their family and friends advance notice and therefore time for intimacy, discussion, and grief before the end. It allows people to experience planned, peaceful dying, and gives the dying the opportunity to say good-bye to family and friends in a loving and meaningful manner. It bonds the dying patient with the surrounding community. Rather than an impulsive act of despair, PAD is a rational act of self-determination based on personal values and spiritual beliefs, and it extends respect and consideration to others.

For example, a study from Oregon, where assisted death is legal, found that family members of patients who died under the law were more peaceful and able to accept their loved ones' dying than comparable families of patients who died naturally but often unexpectedly, or after long, difficult illnesses.[50]

Third, people who commit suicide want to die. In contrast, people who seek PAD would gladly live if they could be relieved of their end-of-life suffering. But because they *are* dying, and nothing can be done to stop that process, it's not a matter of choosing to die but of wanting to control the process of dying.

This distinction is recognized by the Washington State Psychological Association, which has weighed in on whether or not assisted death is a form of emotional or mental disorder:

> Profound   psychological   differences   distinguish

suicide from patient-directed dying. The term suicide is traditionally used to refer to medically well individuals who wish to end their lives because of severe emotional suffering and/or psychiatric disorders. Typically they do not consult with or have the support of others, acting alone, often choosing violent means, and causing suffering to those they leave behind. Mentally competent, terminally ill individuals who wish for a humane and dignified death that is patient-directed, supported by the patient's family and physician, in a situation in which death is inevitable, differ from suicidal, medically well individuals. A person with a terminal illness is going to die even with, or despite, the best medical treatment available. The designation of suicide is disrespectful to individuals with terminal illness who wish to have choice regarding death with dignity, and can be distressing and problematic emotionally, socially, psychologically, and financially for family members and loved ones of dying individuals.[51]

The fact is, physician aid in dying allows dying patients to *avoid* ordinary suicide. Opponents, on the other hand, refer to the act as suicide in order to associate it with the negative emotions associated with ordinary suicide.

The strategic import of this framing was made clear to me when I was driving home one evening in the summer of 2008. Having just returned from a campaign for Washington State's Initiative-1000, otherwise known as the "Death with Dignity Act," I tuned into a radio station that was airing a debate on the proposed act. A listener called in and said, "I'm voting against this initiative because I just can't stand the thought of my dying mother committing suicide!"

That is precisely how opponents want people to react—by having them view it as a sacrilegious act of violence, and an affront to God-given life. A little more discussion with the woman, however, revealed that she was afraid her mother would wander off by herself, or wait until she was alone in her home, and die without anyone else with her. Yet as I have explained, that is not what happens with PAD; the very act of PAD precludes anyone from dying in isolation and secrecy—it opens the dying process to interaction with physician, family, and friends. But by framing the act as suicide, there is only one interpretation that can be made, and that is one of condemnation. Thus the AMA position is based on the faulty premise that for a physician to assist a terminally ill patient to die with dignity is an act of assisting suicide. It is not an act of suicide.

But what about the argument that PAD is fundamentally at odds with the physician's role as a healer? Framing the issue in this manner implies an either/or situation, suggesting doctors should heal *instead of* kill. In other words, it says they *must* heal. Of course, if one had only a choice between killing and healing, one would choose healing, which is why such rhetoric is effective—it leads the listener to feel there is only one moral choice.

Framing the issue as physician-assisted *suicide* rather than physician-assisted *death* shifts perception from the act of dying to the act of aiding in self-killing. Along with this shift comes a shift in the emotional connections the listener makes in evaluating the issue. When we discuss dying, emotions related to grief and compassion are evoked, and we begin to assess the discussion that follows with those emotional cues. But when we discuss suicide or killing, our emotions are more likely to be ones of revulsion, anger, or fear. Listeners who are primed with these emotions are far more likely to be resistant to any ensuing discussion that advocate such an act.

This image of PAD as fundamentally at odds with the practice of medicine and physician ethics depends upon a revised history of actual physician practice, and silence around a practice that every physician is intimately familiar: the manner in which physicians actually do assist patients in dying while maintaining the appearance that they do no such thing.

In the next chapter, we look at why that might be.

CHAPTER 3
FROM HIPPOCRATES TO LASAGNA

FRED DID NOT WANT to die. Fred was a burly, balding, seventy-seven-year-old retired attorney with a no-nonsense attitude he'd picked up from his childhood in the Ohio Rust Belt where people said what was on their minds and let others do the same. Born with "the gift of gab," Fred put his verbal skills to good use and climbed his way out of the working class and into a successful law career in litigation. But his success didn't go to his head. After moving to the West Coast and establishing his career, Fred didn't lose his sensitivity to those who never had life's advantages; he knew how difficult life on the bottom could be, and he did all he could to help those who weren't as fortunate as he had been throughout his life.

I had known Fred for about fifteen years when one day Beverly phoned with bad news—Fred had esophageal cancer. As is commonly the case, it had come on slowly, with weight loss and increasing difficulty swallowing. Fred said he had not felt right for a few weeks, but his wife told me that he had been eating less than usual for at least two months. Eventually, when all his pants were too big for his belt to hold up, he knew it was time to see a doctor.

Fred went to see his primary physician who had him swallow barium, which lit up his esophagus as if he'd swallowed a black light. Almost immediately his doctor saw an illuminated indentation around a portion of the esophagus and knew what it was; he told Fred it looked like cancer. A biopsy confirmed his suspicion, and the family doctor quickly arranged for him to see an oncologist to discuss and begin treatment.

Beverly went with Fred on his first visit to meet the oncologist, along with one of their daughters, who took a day off work to be with him for the visit. The oncologist was polite and almost casual at first, but after a few questions about who Fred was and what he did for a living, the physician's demeanor changed and he became very professional. As Fred listened nervously, the oncologist carefully went over what the X-rays had shown about Fred's cancer, and what the natural course of the disease would be without treatment.

"When you talk about treatment," Beverly asked, "do you mean chemotherapy?"

"Yes, that's right," the doctor answered. "We'll start off with chemotherapy to attack the cancer cells in the esophagus and anywhere else the tumor might have spread"—he seemed to relax a bit more as he explained—"and we'll also use radiation aimed at the tumor."

Fred appeared to be taking it all in very intently, but as with anyone, once the person hears the word "cancer," the words that followed became a wall of sound that his mind couldn't quite penetrate, despite having spent his entire adult life listening and analyzing what other people said. But that was why Beverly and their daughter were there; they would help him negotiate the bewildering road map that lay before him.

"And how long will my dad go through this?" his daughter asked.

"We won't know for sure until we can assess how the cancer cells are responding," he answered, "but you can plan on several months of therapy."

Several months didn't sound like much time at all to Fred and his family, if that's all the time he had left before he died, but several months of being miserable from chemotherapy and radiation was another matter. They knew from the doctor's explanation and what they heard from other cancer patients that those months could be filled with nausea, vomiting, hair loss, anemia, constipation, diarrhea, sores, bleeding, nerve damage, fatigue, and a host of other possible and miserable side effects as his body's good cells were destroyed along with the cancer cells.

"This double approach gives us a good chance of eradicating the cancer," the oncologist optimistically explained, "and after completing the course of chemo and radiation therapy, you'll have surgery to remove the deadened cancer and any other nearby tissue that might harbor any cancer cells that weren't killed."

In other words, Fred's near-eighty-year-old body would be burned, poisoned, and cut into in order to help him live longer if all went well.

Fred listened attentively to the detailed explanation of his forthcoming treatment and interrupted only to ask an occasional technical question.

When the oncologist finished, he looked at Fred and said, "Well, that's about it. Do you have any more questions?"

"Yes," Fred said. "I have one very important question." Fred turned in his chair, looked at his wife, then at his daughter, and then back at the oncologist. "Doctor," he said confidently, "I very much appreciate your excellent description of the planned treatment, and I'm ready to get going with it. But there's one more thing I need to ask you."

"Of course," the doctor responded. "What's that?"

"Well, I expect to get better, and I'm hoping for a cure," Fred began. "But I know that with a disease like this, sooner or later it probably will get the better of me. When that happens, and a cure is no longer possible, at the end, Doctor, will you help me die? Will you help me die peacefully when that time comes?"

"You've come to me to help you live, not die," his doctor responded, clearly disturbed to be presented with the question. "Don't worry; we'll take care of you." Then he bid Fred and his family good-bye and left the room.

Fred knew his doctor would help him all he could but that he might not be willing to do what Fred might ask him to do. Fred didn't want to die, but he knew that when his time came, he wanted his doctor to keep him from suffering any more than was necessary.

Fred began the treatment for his disease, just as the oncologist had described, combining chemotherapy and radiation therapies. He lived about eight miles from the medical center, and every day Beverly cheerfully drove him to and from treatment. A few times Fred was so sick from the chemotherapy, with nausea and vomiting, that he was too weak to go home and had to stay overnight at the medical center. Even on good days he felt weakness over his whole body, but most days when the treatment was over he was able to return home.

Fred became so sick that it was difficult to know which was making him sicker, the treatment or the cancer. At first the tumor was so large he could barely swallow, and eating anything at all just seemed to make him feel worse. But Fred was not a man to give up; he wanted more than anything to live, if only to have one more year with his wife and daughters. So he remained hopeful and got through those rough days and weeks and months, and eventually, after about three months of extensive chemotherapy and radiation, he began to feel some real improvement. He could finally swallow again, but he was still very weak and was not regaining much of the weight he had lost. He hoped that with surgery, his recovery would be complete, or as near complete as he could hope for his age.

But just as he began to feel that at long last the tumor was really shrinking, another round of tests showed that the cancer had spread to other parts of his body, most ominously to his brain. With the tumor no longer localized to his esophagus, surgery was no longer an option. Fred had taken the treatment his doctors had prescribed, but it hadn't worked as well as he or anyone had hoped for. The cancer wasn't disappearing; it was killing him.

Fred went again to talk to his oncologist. The oncologist suggested more, higher-dose chemotherapy with different drugs, saying further treatment most likely would not provide a cure but might offer many more good months of life. He also suggested radiation therapy to the brain in hopes that it might slow the growth of the tumors there. But when Fred asked about complications of further treatment, the oncologist said it would be the same as before—nausea, vomiting, extreme weakness—maybe even more than before because of the newer, stronger medicines they would use.

"It's the best thing we have for you, and it's worth taking the chance," the oncologist added. "Otherwise there's nothing more we can do for you."

Fred sat still in his chair, looking like a convicted man, hair uncombed and shirt hanging in folds around his diminished body. He was mute for at least a minute, while his wife asked questions about how the newer chemotherapy was different and how it would work, whether radiation to the brain would alter Fred's ability to think, and the results the doctor had seen with other patients when the tumor has spread to the brain.

But Fred was having none of it. He was so weak he could hardly keep from slumping over in his chair. He knew, with a lawyer's innate sense, the difference between fact and rhetoric, between desire and common sense. There were no facts to buttress the case for more of the same. He was both judge and jury to his own fate, and he had arrived at his decision.

When his wife had no more questions, and she and the oncologist looked at him, Fred raised his eyes toward his wife and said, "Let's go home."

Fred had had enough dealings with this oncologist to know he wouldn't help him with what he really wanted—to go home and live peacefully for a while and then die without a lot of suffering.

Fred had given it his best shot—he had vomited through extensive chemotherapy and insufferable weakness and fatigue in hopes of what seemed like a reasonable chance to beat the disease. When it became obvious the treatment wasn't working, he went to the finish of the full course of treatment—not because he thought it would help but because he thought he owed it to his wife and family to make a reasonable effort to prolong his life.

But now Fred was ready to stop. He was losing control not only over his disease but over his remaining life. He was dependent on others for almost everything, including help with his personal bodily needs, and this dependence bothered him greatly. Above all, he didn't want to spend the last days, weeks, or months of his life in a hospital, or semisedated at home. So with the help of his family doctor he signed up with a hospice for help in dying at home. The hospice nurses and other caretakers were excellent, and he had no pain. But soon the tumor in his esophagus had grown back, and once again he couldn't swallow solid foods and could take only small amounts of liquids. The hospice nurse suggested he get a feeding tube inserted into his stomach, which would solve the nutritional problem and perhaps give him additional comfortable time.

Fred wasn't interested in any feeding tube. It would only prolong the agony of dying. He knew he had a constitutional right to refuse treatment, and he'd finally reached the point where that was his desire. And although he knew his wife and other family members would continue with their loving care, he didn't want to put them through any more of it. As much as he wanted to live, he knew his body had reached its end.

Through the many months of treatment, Fred had met several physicians—his oncologist, a surgeon who assessed him for possible surgery, radiologists, and many others. They were all specialists, and together they orchestrated all his treatments, wrote his prescriptions, and managed his total care. Yet in all that time, Fred had seen his primary physician of fifteen-plus years only once since first getting the diagnosis and being sent off to the oncologist. He knew his primary physician was the one who knew him best and who would most likely be willing to shepherd him to the end. So he decided to go to him and ask for help in dying peacefully, soon, without waiting until the cancer finally choked off his life.

His wife helped him get outside and seated in the car and then helped him inside the medical office building and into the elevator. This trip, which was once routine, now seemed to Fred like climbing Mount Everest. A nurse put him into a room and began taking off his shirt to get him into an examining gown, but Fred asked her to stop, saying, "I'm only here to talk." So the nurse left, and Fred and his wife waited for their doctor to arrive.

When the doctor entered the room he greeted Fred and his wife, and cheerfully asked the usual, "Hi, Fred, how are you doing?"

Fred first said a little bit about the headaches he was now having, and his weakness and inability to swallow, and then he got to the point. "I just came here to ask you for something."

"Go ahead," said the doctor. "What can I do for you?"

Fred looked first at his wife, then at the doctor, and said softly but firmly, "Doctor, please help me die."

"Wha … what do you mean?" the doctor stammered.

"I mean please give me a medicine I can use, when the time comes, that will put me to sleep and end the suffering," Fred replied.

"But then I would be killing you—you're asking me to be your murderer!" the doctor said incredulously.

"No, I'm not," Fred replied. "I ask you to help me. You're the only physician who can cure my suffering. Please, Doctor, there is only one 'cure' for this cancer; we both know that. Please don't deny me that one comfort."

"I'm sorry," his physician answered. "I wish I could help you. But I can't. I took an oath to do no harm, and helping you die would do just that. I won't play God with life or death." And with those words, the physician said good-bye and left the room.

Fred and Beverly returned home, where Fred remained until his final days, drugged almost to sedation in order to avoid the agonizing pain as the tumors devoured his organs ever so slowly but oh, so surely. Hospice was a big help, but by the time he finally died, Fred suffered in many ways he had wanted to avoid. But he knew one thing for sure: although he was receiving the best possible care, he might have been better off in the hands of an unconventional physician like Dr. Kevorkian; for if he begged a Dr. Kevorkian to end his suffering, he may have shown Fred that one small mercy—a mercy that more caring healers feared to provide.

Why did Fred's physicians readily provide treatments with potential to cause him such great suffering with no guarantee it would prolong his happy life but refuse to help him end that suffering when he was clearly dying? Was it true, as his family physician said, that to do so would be professionally unethical? How could his physician argue that to save lives was *his* job, but to help people to die was *God's* job?

To better understand the answers to these questions, we turn once again to the Greek gods. Asclepius was considered one of the first physicians of the Western world and, like Heracles, the son of a god and a mortal. His father, Apollo, had raped, impregnated, and then killed Asclepius's mortal mother, Coronis, while she was still pregnant with their child. But at the last minute, Apollo, the god of medicine, healing, and knowledge, cut the child from his dead mother and spared his son's life. Asclepius was given to the wise centaur Chiron to raise, and Chiron soon recognized that Asclepius had inherited the gift of healing from his father and set out to train him in the art of medicine.

Asclepius was indeed gifted in the healing arts, and by the time he grew, he had gained fame for helping the lame to walk, giving sight to the blind, and curing the afflicted. But he went too far when he raised a man from the dead; upon hearing of that achievement, the gods' approval turned to rage. How dare a demigod undermine the rule of the gods by restoring life to the dead? Zeus, king of the gods, was outraged, as was his brother, Hades, lord of the underworld. Hades was furious to think that no more dead spirits would come to the underworld if physicians could so easily raise the dead and return them to live on earth, and he and his powerful brother knew something had to be done about Apollo's impudent son.

What Asclepius had done was an unpardonable sin, and one that set a very dangerous precedent undermining the rule of the gods. He had committed hubris, or an act of arrogance, because only the gods could shape the destiny of mortals; only they controlled life and death. Asclepius had to be stopped—and more importantly, a lesson had to be made of his hubris so that no one dared replicate his audacious act. Never one to let bygones be bygones, the enraged Zeus crashed through the heavens and struck Asclepius dead with a thunderbolt. Then to be sure all in the universe knew what fate befell any mortal who played as a god, he hurled the body of Asclepius into the heavens where it remains to this day, as the constellation Ophiuchus, "the serpent bearer."

It's in God's Hands

The Hippocratic physicians who descended from Asclepius taught that illness is due to natural bodily malfunction rather than supernatural or divine causes. But most of the Hippocratic physicians continued to believe in the influence of the gods over matters of life and death. That is, although illnesses could be explained by natural mechanisms, the gods influenced these natural phenomena. And, "fate," or "the will of the gods" remained, by and large, the answer to the question of how and when mortals die.

Over the millennia the principle of "the will of the gods" became, within the monotheistic religions of the Western world, "the will of God." Through the Middle Ages and beyond, the Christian church reinforced the principle of divine control over life and death, while accommodating naturalist-based physicians by treating them as agents of God in the struggle against evil. This view has permeated Western worldviews on health and healing in complex and subtle ways. Most Americans view serious illness and death as somehow divinely ordained, and this belief in many cases provides a certain solace that helps people accept what they cannot themselves control.

When I was a medical intern in the state of Michigan, I discovered just how powerful this belief system can be in helping patients and their families cope with suffering. It was my first patient rotation, and I was assigned to a pediatric service in a general hospital. Although I was seriously considering going into pediatrics as a specialty, I often found working with sick kids distressing because it was difficult to see them suffering.

One of the children on "my service" was a lovely six-year-old little girl named Jessie, who was suffering from a rare blood disease. Although there are better treatments today, at that time the only treatment—a blood transfusion—was relatively ineffectual. I learned from reading the chart that she would probably die within a few weeks, if not sooner.

Jessie had long, curly dark hair, and she always clung to a septic-looking, threadbare baby doll. No matter how hard I tried to make her laugh, Jessie seemed unable to produce a smile. Instead, she had a habit of looking away whenever I approached her bedside, and this habit bothered me a great deal. I knew it wasn't just me she didn't want to see, as she never looked at the other doctors either, and when we asked her questions, she just looked at her mother for an answer. The mother, who slept nights on a couch in the nearby "family room," was ever-present and ministering through the day to her daughter's requests for water or other needs.

One morning while making our rounds, the attending pediatrician explained that while Jessie's condition was worsening, another blood transfusion would give her body more time to fight the disease. When the pediatrician asked the mother if it was all right to go ahead with another transfusion, the mother responded, "It's all in God's hands. Do what God tells you to do."

Jessie got her transfusion, and according to her mother she felt somewhat better, though Jessie still would not look us in the eye or talk to us directly.

But within a week it was clear to all the medical staff that she was now worse than before the last transfusion. The options for Jessie were exhausted, despite our best efforts. At a meeting at which the entire medical staff discussed difficult cases, Jessie's case was raised. The overwhelming opinion was that we should discharge Jessie to die in the comfort of her own home.

When we got to Jessie's room on our rounds, I was the last one in the door, and I didn't want to look at her, knowing that her fate had been determined—there was nothing we could possibly do to cure her. The pediatrician was as gentle as he could be, but he soon came to the point. He acknowledged that the transfusions had made Jessie feel better for a few days, but he explained that they weren't stopping the disease. He continued to tell her and her family that although we would give Jessie another transfusion if she wanted it, it would be best to let Jessie go home where she would be more comfortable.

"Is that all right with you?" the pediatrician asked the mother.

"It's in God's hands. If he wants Jessie to go home, we'll take her home."

Jessie went home, where she died surrounded by her family. But for me, that explanation was troubling because to me it was not God who wanted her sent home but a medical establishment that could do nothing—at that time—to save her.

There may not be a single physician practicing today who has not heard a patient state the belief that life is in God's hands. The belief of divine control over human life, although not universally held, is deeply imbedded in all religiously based cultures, as it is in ours. For that reason, physicians are often accused of "playing God," and even viewing themselves as godlike, for the very fact that they do save lives. Yet saving lives is no longer considered trespassing on the territory of the gods, as it was in the time of

Asclepius, because as Judea-Christianity took root in the Western philosophical tradition, humans became viewed as created in the image of God. Hence, to save lives is to serve God. But *to take* lives continues to be viewed as interfering with the will of God because with the biblical prohibition of "Thou shalt not kill," taking a life for any reason can be viewed as violating a commandment of God. When Fred asked his physician to help him die, his physician responded that he couldn't play God with life and death. Just as Jessie's mother viewed her death as in God's hands, for Fred's physician, to help Fred die was usurping the divine role of God.

But if they view themselves as servants of God, and the will of God is for their patient to die, why do physicians so resist the thought of providing their patients a less painful death by ending their suffering? To better understand the answer to that question, we turn now to a closer look at the Hippocratic Oath.

The Hippocratic Oath

"Doctors take an oath not to kill their patients," began the pro-life speaker at a political rally, "and mercy killing is breaking that oath."

The speaker was expressing a commonly held belief that upon graduating from medical school, graduates take an oath that they "will do no harm," nor give any drug to a patient that will hasten death. What the speaker was undoubtedly referring to is the Hippocratic Oath—which medical schools began phasing out as far back as the late-nineteenth century, when the ancient pledge proved inadequate for the realities of modern medicine.

Almost everyone knows about the Hippocratic Oath and assumes that all physicians swear by it when graduating from medical school. But contrary to popular belief, very few medical students today take the Hippocratic Oath because most modern medical schools either do not require it, or they substitute a more modern version.

Yet those who oppose physician-assisted dying (PAD) continue to use the Hippocratic Oath to support their contention that physicians are sworn not to help people to die. A closer look at Hippocrates and the oath suggests, however, that opponents might do better to rethink using both the oath, and its purported author, to support any right-to-life position.

Hippocrates was an ancient Greek physician, considered the father of Western medicine, who lived from approximately 460–370 BC. Two decades of his life were spent in prison, where he had been banished for his opposition to the Greek government. It was during his years of imprisonment that he wrote a number of medical treatises, although whether he was the actual author of the oath that bears his name is a matter of speculation. We simply do not know who wrote the Hippocratic Oath.

What we do know is that the earliest known manuscript of the oath is from at least thirteen hundred years after Hippocrates's other writings. As with most any writing that has survived for so many centuries, the oath has been revised numerous times through the ages. Given that it wasn't until the first century AD that the oath was even mentioned, few if any scholars today believe the oath that bears his name was written by Hippocrates, but that minor detail does little to diminish the importance of either the great scholar's contributions to medicine, or the significance of the oath as a foundation by which medical ethics have developed. By calling on physicians to be honorable, to keep the confidence of their patients, not to have sexual relations or other conflicting interests with their patients, and to put the needs and concerns of their patients first and foremost in their care, the Hippocratic Oath and its many variations have served as a symbolic code by which physicians will ideally conduct themselves.

But by far the most important use of the Hippocratic Oath in contemporary times is as a cudgel against those who would assist patients in dying. The oath, which also admonishes physicians to "give no deadly poison," is cited by opponents as the bedrock principle of medical ethics, and a transcendent and immemorial injunction against physician-assisted dying. But according to most prominent medical historians, the oath was influenced by Pythagorean mystics who believed in the transmigration of souls (reincarnation as humans, animals, or natural objects), alchemy, and pentagrams.

The Pythagoreans were far more influential to occultists than to contemporary fundamentalist Christians, yet they did oppose abortion and euthanasia. In that regard, however, their views on the topic were among the minority for their time; many other Greek physicians of the time accepted these practices.

As leading historian Darrel W. Amundsen put it, the Hippocratic Oath's prohibitions against abortion and euthanasia, "are inconsistent with values expressed by the majority of sources and atypical of the realities of ancient medical practice."[52] With the notable exception of the Hippocratic Oath, not a single Hippocratic writer voices opposition to voluntary euthanasia, and some medical historians have gone so far as to say that Hippocrates himself practiced abortions and assisted death on occasion.[53]

Among all physician oaths, the Hippocratic Oath is perhaps the most ironic for opponents of PAD to point to in supporting right-to-life arguments. Consider the very first statement of the Hippocratic Oath: "I swear, by Apollo physician and Asclepius and Hygeia and Panaceia and all the other gods and goddesses …"

In other words, the Hippocratic Oath is a *pagan* oath! Those who quote from the oath to condemn PAD are making an argument that an oath to pagan gods must be honored. Yet, were the minority of graduating medical students who do take the Hippocratic Oath to literally honor it, they would also be compelled to share their income with their teachers, teach their craft to only males (and without pay), and never use the knife—which is to say, perform no surgery. A very impractical oath, indeed, but in its day it provided an important ethical code by which physicians held themselves and their colleagues to account.

But what of the oath's proscription to "give no deadly poison"? First, let us consider how poisons are defined. Classifying substances as medicines, drugs, toxins, poisons, or nutrients is never an easy process. For one thing, many, if not all, medicines are derived from substances that in certain doses, forms, contexts, or uses can be toxic or deadly. For another, how a substance is viewed by the one using it, administering it, selling it, and producing it contributes to how it is valued.

Take, for example, substances classed as stimulants. Coffee beans, cacao, and many plant leaves (such as teas) contain low to high levels of caffeine and can be considered nutritional, medicinal, or merely pleasurable. Other stimulants, such as amphetamines, may be considered deadly and addictive drugs, and those who produce, sell, and use them may be viewed as criminals or addicts. These same amphetamines, when prescribed by a physician to a hyperactive child and administered by a parent or guardian, may be considered medication.

Similarly, alcohol was used in Hippocrates's time as a common medication for a range of ailments, and its nutritive value and social role have a long and notable history. Yet few substances have killed as many as alcohol has. Is it an elixir of the gods, or a deadly poison? The answer lies in how the substance is used, to whom it is administered, and the meanings that are attached to it. Understanding these variables that determine how a substance is defined may help us understand the origins of the Hippocratic Oath's proscription against administering deadly poisons.

The admonition to physicians to "give no deadly poison" is cited by opponents of physician-assisted death as an unambiguous principle of medical ethics. But the admonition to "give no deadly poison" may have been one of the profession's first public-relations gambits. The physicians of the time had few medicaments of any therapeutic benefit by today's standards, but they did have one substance that was very powerful and effective—poisons. In all likelihood, the Hippocratic physicians did occasionally use these substances as a last desperate attempt to arrest the disease—similar to how high doses of chemotherapy are used today to attack cancer cells while knowing they will attack good cells as well.

They also used poisons occasionally at the urging of dying patients, to help them die, a practice for which they were criticized by a minority of others. Knowledge of this latter practice may well have tarnished the reputation of the Hippocratic physicians who competed with several other types of healers at the time. There was a real fear that the treatment a doctor administered could kill as much as heal because many patients did die at the hands of the physician. Moreover, with beliefs in sorcery still strong, anyone who possessed specialized knowledge of ethnopharmacology—the use of plants as medicines—was a potential poisoner. For this reason, some physicians were suspected to have poisoned patients at the request of others, for money or another motive. Thus, the "give no deadly poison" clause of the oath provided reassurance to the populace that the physician had vowed not to engage in sorcery or other evildoing. As one physician of the time, Aulus Cornelius Celsus, said, "For it is the part of a prudent man not to risk the appearance of having killed one whose lot is but to die."[54]

Because so many medications are indeed deadly, not only through overdoses but from "side effects" that cause strokes, heart attacks, addiction, suicidal ideation, organ damage, hypertension, pulmonary disorders, miscarriage, and other harmful reactions, physicians cannot possibly treat their patients with modern pharmaceuticals without risking delivering a "deadly poison." Just as in Hippocrates's time, when diseases were often treated with known poisons that in skilled hands could provide sufficient dosage to heal but not kill the patient, or they were sedated with alcohol that was known to be deadly to some patients but calming to others, the administration of medicine by its very nature requires providing patients with potentially deadly poisons.

Yet some physicians did intentionally administer poisons to facilitate death during Hippocrates's time, or they refrained from administering medication and treatment. In a treatise attributed to Hippocrates and entitled simply "The Art," the author advises for the purpose of physicians: "In general terms, it is to do away with the sufferings of the sick, to lessen the violence of their diseases, and to refuse to treat those who are overmastered by their disease, realizing that in such cases medicine is powerless."[55]

The first two parts of this passage, "to do away with the sufferings of the sick" and "to lessen the violence of their diseases," speak to the attitude of acting for the benefit of patients that makes the Hippocratic writings and the Hippocratic Oath universally admired. But what should we make of the enigmatic statement, "refuse to treat those who are overmastered by their disease"? Why would physicians refuse to help those who were dying? Granted, by our modern standards the medications of the ancients were relatively powerless to arrest or reverse fatal illnesses, but in the same sense it could be argued that they were equally powerless for all patients, not just those who were dying. Even so, the ancient physicians had remedies and methods to instill hope, alleviate pain, and soothe the minds of ill patients, so why practice any differently with patients who are dying? Why should they abandon their patients in their time of greatest need?

The admonition to not attend dying patients derived in part from a desire not to increase the agony of patients with therapy that at best might only prolong the dying process, an attitude many modern physicians would do well to accept. In order to avoid treating dying patients, the Hippocratic physicians withdrew from their patients when they could no longer cure them. But they had another, more practical concern about attending a dying patient: the inevitable death might appear to be caused by the physician regardless of what treatment he was giving, thereby tainting his reputation. Therefore, care of the dying was left to families or the ancient equivalent of nurses. By this ancient practice physicians established dying as outside of their business—as something separate from living and illness.

This practice foreshadowed the strong tendency of physicians today to disengage from dying patients for whom there are no medical treatments remotely likely to cure or extend life, and specifically to avoid any appearance of helping them die through medical means. What's still important to physicians today is not to be administering or undertaking a medicine or any treatment when the patient is next to his final breath, as the doctor's presence may signal a cause-and-effect relationship to observers. So for all but a dedicated few physicians, it is considered best for the doctor to be out of the patient's room when the end is imminent. This is a Hippocratic-based modern version of abandonment; the physician may attend the patient throughout the disease, but once the disease—and patient—has reached the end, physicians will leave patients to meet the end without a doctor by their side.

Absent at the End

This absence of the physician at the scene of death is a common theme in movies of death, beginning with the very first movies to address the topic. For example, in the 1939 movie *Dark Victory*, Bette Davis plays heiress Judith Traherne, a devil-may-care socialite who revels in life's pleasures. But when she begins having blinding headaches and dizzy spells, she sees a brain specialist who discovers she has a brain tumor and will die—painlessly but quickly—within the year. Like Dr. Morrison in the 1948 film *An Act of Murder*, the physician opts to conceal the dire prognosis from his patient so that she might enjoy what little time she has left. A romance between doctor and patient ensues, and again like the later film *An Act of Murder*, the dying woman discovers the truth. But here the similarities between the two films end, as the dying woman of *Dark Victory* chooses to live rather than die. And live she does, until she realizes (with the help of Humphrey Bogart, playing a lovelorn stable hand) that her dying days would best be spent with the doctor she truly loves. She returns to him, spending her final days tending to their home, and her final hours tending to her garden, until she realizes the end has come. Then, with the doctor away delivering a paper on his latest medical breakthrough, she ascends the stairs and lies down upon her bed to die alone and at peace, her death natural and painless.

The absence of physicians from their patients' death scenes are notable in both movies. The doctors have personal as well as professional relationships with their patients, suggesting a deep concern for their well-being. In both movies, the doctors conceal the truth from their patients, and in both movies, although they prescribe medicines and manage their patients' suffering to the best of their ability, when the illnesses become most dire, the doctors are far away. By removing the doctors from these death scenes, they remain untarnished by the grim reality of death they can't prevent. In 1939's *Dark Victory*, the physician cannot be faulted for his failure to keep his patient alive because he wasn't even there when death arrived. In his company and care, she lived; in his absence, she died. But a decade later, in the 1948 *An Act of Murder*, the physician had prescribed the lethal pills, unaware his patient took them to end her life. Later making it clear that he opposed "mercy killing" for any reason, the physician's culpability in his patient's death was cleared. He may have prescribed the "deadly poison," but he had nothing to do with his patient's final act in taking the fatal dose.

Life does indeed imitate art, but the absence of physicians from their patients' bedside when they are dying is not necessarily a reflection of physician indifference. Patients who ask their physicians to help them die should understand the desire of their doctors to avoid the *appearance* of helping, even when the physician may feel it would be better for the patient if the doctor actually could help. Doctors do not want to abandon their patients, but even more so, they do not want to be associated with assisted dying—they want to give their patients a sense of hope they will not die. And while some near-saintly physicians do follow their patients to the very end, or at least as close to the end as possible, those who do are a small minority. And with more patients opting to die outside the hospital, even these few physicians often find it impossible to be there for their patients when they do die because the medical system now makes house calls nearly impossible for physicians who must be ever-present in the clinical setting and see increasingly large numbers of patients every day.

Thus, patients often underestimate the tension that physicians face in wanting to help their patients but not wanting to appear to be angels of death. But few physicians realize how this more pressing need to not be associated with death is one way in which they continue to follow the teachings of Hippocrates. While modern physicians themselves are very unlikely to take the Hippocratic Oath, or to view their own practices as related to Hippocrates's writings, the public imagination—and arguments against PAD—persist in viewing the ancient medical traditions of Hippocrates as the primary foundation on which medical ethics are based. In doing so, however, they rarely consider the entirety of the ancient philosopher's teachings, or the text of the oath itself. Instead, those who point to the Hippocratic Oath as a defense against PAD virtually always rely on the "do no harm," and "deadly poisons" clauses as the sole ethical guidepost by which to evaluate a physician's practice, while ignoring the rest of the oath—or other ethical codes or values that guide physicians in their practice.

Hippocratic Oath Redux

Despite the reality that physicians of ancient times commonly refrained from treating the dying or hastened their death by administering deadly doses of medication—knowingly or in keeping with standard medical practice of the time—opponents of PAD commonly use the "give no deadly poison" clause as the single most powerful ethical guideline by which the conduct of physicians should be evaluated. But in doing so, they display the common facility of rhetoricians of quoting selectively from a tract while disregarding parts unfavorable to their purpose; as I have previously pointed out, the oath also admonishes physicians not to perform surgery and to only train male students. If modern physicians were held to all the instructions of the Hippocratic

Oath, virtually none today would pass muster, and few could engage in the practice of modern medicine.

It is for this reason that graduating medical students take any one of a number of differing oaths, or none at all. One of these was released in 1995 by the National Catholic Bioethics Center, which proposed restating the Hippocratic Oath to include, "I will maintain the utmost respect for every human life from fertilization to natural death."[56] This is a remarkable statement in light of the fact that modern medicine prevents natural death and prolongs life through artificial means!

But among the most significant variations on the Hippocratic Oath is the Declaration of Geneva. Just as fears of ancient physicians using their esoteric knowledge of medicines to poison their patients prompted the "use no deadly poisons" provision of the Hippocratic Oath, in the wake of World War II, it was discovered that Nazi physicians had cooperated in some of the most heinous crimes imaginable against prisoners of the concentration camps, including torture and euthanasia. To ensure that the medical profession not be tainted by the stigma of these atrocities, in 1948 the World Medical Association adopted the "Declaration of Geneva" and later amended it in 2006.[57] The concern of the drafters of the declaration was not that physicians play no role in assisted death but that they not violate human rights. The Declaration includes the following:

1948: The health and life of my patient will be my first consideration. I will maintain the utmost respect for human life; from the time of its conception, even under threat, I will not use my medical knowledge contrary to the laws of humanity.

2006: The health of my patient will be my first consideration. I will maintain the utmost respect for human life. I will not use my medical knowledge to violate human rights and civil liberties, even under threat.

As the oath and its changes make clear, the concern of the World Medical Association was not to advocate a right-to-life approach to medical care but to ensure that physicians do not abuse or misuse their skills toward inhumane ends. Importantly, by changing the pledge from "The health *and life* of my patient will be my first consideration"[58] to "the health of my patient will be my first consideration," the association signaled that prolonging life for life's sake was not necessarily an ethical obligation of the global physician. But what about the American physician? Does the Declaration of Geneva have any weight at all in the US medical profession?

While few medical schools use the Hippocratic Oath today, and about one quarter write their own oaths, many medical schools in the United States do require their graduates to take the Geneva Declaration as their oath, in the expectation that these new physicians take their role as global citizens seriously.

But perhaps the most common oath that newly minted physicians take in the United States today is the oddly named "Oath of Lasagna." Louis Lasagna was a Tufts University professor of medicine who in 1964 called for an international competition to update the Hippocratic Oath. While little is known about the outcome of the competition, his own contribution has become widely popular in American medical schools. The Lasagna Oath is often used by opponents of PAD as evidence that the practice has been explicitly condemned by the following statement: "If it is given me to save a life, all thanks. But it may also be within my power to take a life; this awesome responsibility must be faced with great humbleness and awareness of my own frailty. Above all, I must not play at God."

Here we must emphasize the import of interpretation. The Lasagna Oath does clearly call for physicians to "not play God," and when faced with the prospect of taking a life, to approach the matter with humility and a keen awareness of one's responsibility. But it does not say that the physician ought not to assist the dying patient end his or her suffering; it merely says not to do so lightly. More to the point, another provision of the Lasagna oath bears reflection: I will apply, for the benefit of the sick, all measures

[that] are required, avoiding those twin traps of overtreatment and therapeutic nihilism."

For the physician to reject assisted death in favor of extending life and suffering through artificial means would clearly constitute overtreatment if not therapeutic nihilism. Lasagna himself recognized the moral imperatives facing physicians in light of the rapid changes that science and technology bring to medicine, leading to new questions of what it means to treat the dying: "The very act of dying has been so altered in recent centuries as to necessitate a reexamination of our system of moral and societal values. Even euthanasia, so long barred from ethical and legal discussions, is now under scrutiny by many thoughtful scientists and laymen. A review of the past shows that a rigid, dogmatic attitude toward death is historically, scientifically, and morally indefensible."[59]

Nevertheless, although contemporary physicians rarely take an oath prohibiting their participation in PAD, oaths have far less influence on a physician's actual behavior than does their professional code of ethics. And here is where opponents of PAD have a more sound institutional footing on which to condemn it and where I argue that physicians themselves have created their resistance to openly advocating the legalization of PAD—despite continuing to engage in the practice more covertly. Turning now to the AMA, we consider how physicians learn to conform to the expectations of their peers.

CHAPTER 4
PHYSICIAN, HEAL THY PATIENT

FEW EXPERIENCES IN LIFE are as intimate and uncertain as the illness experience. When our health is disturbed, we turn to our physicians and the medical system for explanation and cure. As anthropologist and psychiatrist Arthur Kleinman has written, the patient views the entire medical system as a healing system.[60] The physician, in the eyes of the patient, is at the helm of this healing system, acting primarily as a healer who is charged with doing everything possible to restore the patient's health. Thus, the core relationship in clinical care is between the physician and patient; in order to effectively communicate and share the intimacies of the illness experience, the patient must trust the physician will do his or her utmost to heal the patient. But a fundamental tension between patient and healer is that very often each has very different ideas of what constitutes "healing." This tension is reflected in the distinction between illness and disease.

Although we often talk about illness and disease interchangeably, social scientists distinguish between the two. Disease refers more specifically to the biological disorder that is causing the patient's health problem, and illness is the patient's experience of a health concern. Illness can subsume not just the physical discomforts and disabilities that are experienced when the body is not functioning properly but also the psychological and social impacts that accompany a health problem. For example, a person whose cancer has advanced to a late stage has a very serious disease. But if that person has been relatively symptom free and has not been diagnosed or treated until he or she is aware of the disease, the patient's health may be endangered, but he or she is not ill. Similarly, someone who has aches and pains throughout his or her body may have nothing physically wrong, but the person's suffering may be very real. It is fair to say that person not have a disease but is suffering from an illness. Moreover, the illness experience affects not just the patient's well-being but the patient's primary relationships, including caregivers, dependents, and even employers. The illness experience, then, is distinct from the disease process; though the two often correspond and the disease may cause very predictable signs and symptoms, one is the objective disorder the physician attempts to diagnose and cure, and the other is the subjective experience the patient seeks to be healed from.

It follows then that throughout the patient/healer interaction, the patient has expectations that the physician will alleviate their suffering, while the physician views her or his role as to heal illness but cure disease. When the disease has advanced to such a stage that the patient is dying, alleviating pain and discomfort—however inadequately—may well be the only way the physician can perceive being able to successfully carry out the healing role—by healing the suffering of the illness, despite being unable to cure the disease that is bringing on such suffering.

From the perspective of the patient, however, there is often little distinction between curing and healing, or between illness and disease. The patient more likely may view the doctor's healing role as extending help with dying—because to the patient who is suffering from the ultimate "illness experience," if death is the only way to reverse the illness experience, facilitating that death may be viewed as consistent with the physician's role as healer, even if the physician does not see healing as extending quite so far.

But what does it mean to heal? First, one cannot understate the professional role of healing for physicians. From long before the time of Hippocrates, physicians were healers, and any nonhealing activity a physician performed ran the risk of diminishing the healing role. This view is the basis of the Hippocratic dictum, "Do not attend the patient who is overmastered by his disease." The patient overmastered by his disease cannot be healed, and as previously discussed, to associate too closely with the dying could jeopardize the physician were he associated with the death. This dictum has been so entrenched in medical training and practice that the first US hospitals would not even admit dying patients![61] As a consequence of this longstanding caution to avoid dying patients, and the prominence of the view of the physician as exclusively a healer, many physicians today view themselves as healers and carry out their healing role by treating, which in modern times means attempting to cure or contain the biophysical disease. By definition, healers treat, or heal, and to help shorten a long-drawn-out life is, in this line of thinking, to be an antihealer, or apostate. As one physician opponent of PAD put it, helping patients die "seriously distorts the healing relationship."[62]

Yet this argument rests more on professional concerns than on concerns for the patient. The "role of the healer" dictum all too often leads physicians to pursue healing in the form of curative medicine—such as drugs, operations, or irradiation—as long as possible, which is frequently to the determinant of adequate comfort care.

This quest to heal is powerfully portrayed in the 2001 film *Wit* starring Emma Thompson as a professor of English who is diagnosed with Stage IV ovarian cancer. Her only hope, her doctor tells her, is for an experimental chemotherapy regime that is very powerful but might prove effective. She agrees to the treatment and is admitted to a hospital for a series of increasingly powerful doses of chemotherapy. The treatment leaves her very ill and proves futile. Eventually, it becomes clear the physicians treating her do not see her as a human but as a case of cancer they hope to conquer. Her comfort is of no concern to them; treating her cancer is their only objective, one they persist in pursuing despite her eventual desire to just die in peace. When her nurse discusses whether she wants a do-not-resuscitate (DNR) order placed in her chart, she agrees, only to have the physicians ignore the order and frantically try to revive her when she goes into cardiac arrest. The dramatic conflict between the nurse attempting to honor the patient's wishes to die and the physicians hoping to resuscitate her in order to continue treating the cancer, demonstrates just how powerful the healing role can be to physicians. Moreover, just as in the movie *Wit*, it was not until the nurse raised the issue that the patient was given the option of a DNR order, in the real world physicians do not always behave differently.

One reason they do not behave differently is because in the past, as we have seen, physicians have been educated and socialized into viewing their role as one of healing and curing; to allow a patient to die is thus viewed by physicians, however subliminally, as a failure on their part.

So why is the push for less-prolonged, more-peaceful dying more prominent or urgent now? If we human beings have put up with end-of-life suffering from time immemorial, why should we change now? There are those who revile the very mention of doctor-patient discussions about end-of-life care, saying it leads to Godless killing. Are they right to say we should accept our fate and not clamor for choice in the matter? If great-grandpa took his pneumonia like a man, choking on his secretions for the last few days of his life, why should we have it any easier? Because things have changed, that's why.

We Die Differently—Bertha

When Louis Lasagna noted fifty years ago that the act of dying had been altered in recent centuries, he probably could not have imagined the speed with which it would be altered in the fifty years to follow. Science and technology advance at an exponential rate, and the decades that followed the computer revolution have had an unimaginable impact on reducing mortality and extending life. To grasp the implications of these changes in medical science, consider the following two cases from my own medical career.

The first "real live" patient I had was when I was a medical student in Philadelphia in 1959. I was working at the Hospital of the University of Pennsylvania, and my task was to interview a fifty-eight-year-old woman named Bertha who, to me at least, seemed bigger than life. In medical parlance, my job was to "take her history."

When I first approached my patient's bedside, dressed in shirt and tie but most notably not wearing a white coat marking me as a physician, I must have had the look of a five-year-old walking into kindergarten for the first time.

"Hi, are you Bertha?" I asked her, doing my best not to let on I had never taken a patient's history before.

"What do you want?" she answered, clearly in no mood for my company.

"My name's Tom," I told her, "and I'm a medical student."

"I thought so," Bertha said, looking the other way. "You're young enough to be my son."

My mood deflated as I realized that as proud as I was to be a medical student, my patient apparently just saw me as a kid.

"Well, do you mind if I ask you some questions?" I asked, looking down at my clipboard with its two sheets of questions covering what seemed to me to be about every conceivable aspect of Bertha's life.

"What do you want to ask me?" She was dressed in a hospital gown, like all the other patients, and sitting up in her bed, which was halfway to the back of a ward of about thirty-two patients, lined up sixteen on a side, separated only by thin, sliding curtains. She looked to be of normal height and weight for her age, wore no makeup, and her long, wavy hair was unkempt. And she had a dressing over an area about three inches long on her forehead.

"Well," I said, looking at my clipboard, "what has brought you here to the hospital?"

"You don't have to go through everything on that clipboard, do you?" Bertha asked, her eyes widening with what I assumed was fright.

I knew I was getting nowhere with Bertha, so I pleaded for sympathy, explaining that med school required me to take patient histories.

"Aren't you a little young for this?" she asked me.

I began to protest that I was quite old enough, but my efforts to assure her of my maturity seemed to humor more than reassure her. But that was all that it took to establish some rapport. For Bertha was soon cooperative, however reluctantly. She told me she was from South Philadelphia, where she lived in a low-income "row house" with her daughter and an eight-year-old grandson whose father had died in a car crash several years ago. Over the next forty-five minutes we talked and even exchanged a few laughs while I, with my crib sheet, was able to delve into the mysteries of her medical problems.

"I have a valve in my heart that won't open up," she explained, "and the blood can't get out of my heart."

I quickly jotted down her explanation, being sure to translate it into the language of my profession. I asked her some more questions and learned that she'd had episodes of dizziness and several "blackout spells," during which she sometimes fell and woke up on the floor. She also became very short of breath just walking up one flight of stairs and generally lacked energy for most physical chores.

In short, I learned Bertha had *aortic stenosis*, which is a deterioration of the valve that opens to let blood out of the heart when it beats, and closes between beats to stop blood from falling back into the heart between beats. For some reason, Bertha's aortic valve had scarred and thickened so much it only opened about a fifth or less as wide as normal, and this meant she wasn't getting enough blood to her body for most activities, particularly physical exertion. And occasionally, if Bertha moved too quickly and the little trickle of blood getting out of her heart went mostly to her muscles, other areas of her body didn't get their usual share. When her brain got shortchanged this way, Bertha fainted. That's what got her into the hospital—she had fallen going up the outside steps to her home, leaving an ugly, two-inch-long gash on the side of her forehead. A neighbor took her to the hospital, and after stitching the wound the emergency room doctor examined her more thoroughly and heard a very loud heart murmur. She was then admitted to the hospital two days before I saw her. In 1959 there was no open-heart surgery for her problem, and the only drug they had for her was digitalis, which was intended to make her heart beat all the harder to get more blood through the diseased valve. Unfortunately, digitalis was largely ineffective, but it was all the science we had back then to help her.

I had no need to see Bertha again, having completed my interview and written up my report, but this first medical encounter, informal as it may have been, bored into me as an emotionally important landmark. I wanted to see Bertha again, to acknowledge the impact our conversation had had on me as a novice in the field of medicine. I had intruded on her in her sickbed, a total stranger young enough to be her own child, and though a bit rough at first, she treated me kindly and shared a private part of her life with me—her damaged body. That may well be what patients do with doctors, but still, the fact that she had let her guard down and opened up to me helped me realize that, routine as it may be for a doctor to take a patient history, it is not routine for a patient to give it.

As it happened, I passed by the hospital the next day, so I decided to drop in to see Bertha. It was about five p.m. on a cold December day when I entered the dimly lit Ward B, the women's ward. As I walked one-by-one past other patients sitting in or next to their beds, I imagined that Bertha had warned them all about me, and so I looked only ahead to where I had been just the day before. I didn't want them to realize that I was that "young" medical student whom Bertha had humbled the day before.

But, curiously, I couldn't find Bertha. The bed she had been in was vacant, so I assumed she had been discharged and gone home. I had been standing at the foot of her bed for a few moments when the patient in the next bed said, "Too bad. Too bad about Bertha."

"What do you mean, 'too bad'?" I asked, surprised and bewildered.

"Well, she died so suddenly," she said. "There was nothing they could do for her."

"*She died?*" I gasped. I couldn't believe it. She was sick, I knew, but still so alive.

"Yes, she was just lying in bed when I heard her moan. At first I didn't think anything of it, but when she just lay there without moving I called to her. She didn't say nothing. I thought it was none of my business to try to talk to her, and she just lay there all still. About ten minutes later, when one of the nurses came by I said she should check on Bertha to see if she was all right. She did, and all of a sudden the nurse gasped, and then pulled the sheet up over Bertha's face and closed the curtains around her bed. They say she died suddenly in her sleep, but I know she wasn't sleeping just before she died."

To say this was a shock to me would be an understatement. Just the day before, Bertha had taught me how to take a medical history, and now she was teaching me how to handle a patient's death. A second transformative medical experience a day after the first was more than I wanted, especially this one. And what was I doing there, anyway?

I walked back out of the ward, looking only at the floor, easing my way out toward the street and normal life. But I had to pass through the nurses' station, and there I saw the medical resident who the day before had assigned me to interview Bertha and told me where to find her. He caught my eye, so I went over to where he was leaning over a medical chart, and asked, "What happened to Bertha?"

"Sudden cardiac death," he said. "Either cardiac standstill or ventricular fibrillation, secondary to aortic stenosis," he added. "That's what often happens."

That was it. She was dead, either because her heart simply stopped or because it went so fast it was effectively pumping no blood. But whatever caused her death, Bertha never knew what happened. It was that sudden.

We Die Differently—Charles

Thirty years later, and I was still learning from my patients about how it is we die. It was a pleasant, sunny Saturday morning in 1989 when I went in to the hospital to make the rounds of my patients. The nerves I'd felt before meeting Bertha were long behind me; I was now a seasoned and successful cardiologist, well accustomed to talking with my patients.

I came to a room occupied by a man I had known for about seven or eight years; his name was Charles, and he was eighty-six years old. When I had first met Charles he was having increasing difficulty with aortic stenosis, the very same condition that had killed Bertha thirty years before. The major valve in Charles's heart that controlled the blood flowing out of it and into his body had deteriorated. He was not passing out from fainting spells, as Bertha had, but he frequently felt lightheaded and couldn't walk up a flight of stairs without stopping about every third step. Although surgery is always risky for a man in his late-seventies, replacing the diseased valve with an artificial valve by then had become standard treatment. So, because he was in otherwise good health, Charles had the operation. Although going through open-heart surgery is no picnic, after a short recovery, he was once again walking without dizzy spells and living a life satisfactory to him.

But Charles's heart was far from healthy; although the artificial valve was working well, years of strenuous pumping to force the blood through the narrowed valve had weakened the heart muscle itself. Although the operation gave him three or four good years he otherwise would not have had, after those few years the shortness of breath returned, and his activities once again became limited. We treated him for congestive heart failure, with some success, but doing so required ever-increasing doses of more and stronger medicines. Charles never complained throughout his ordeal, even after reaching the point where he could no longer walk and had to sleep sitting up to avoid breathlessness. He had been admitted to the hospital two days before to see if we couldn't find a better combination of drugs to ease his breathlessness.

Now, standing outside his room in the Intensive Care Unit on a Saturday morning looking at his medical chart, I was surprised and dismayed to read that he had had a cardiac arrest in the middle of the night. The staff on-call gave him an electrical shock to restart his heart, and although his blood pressure was now dangerously low, he had survived the event. I walked into his room to find him bolt upright, with a grayish hew across his well-aged face. He turned his head of thinned white hair toward me and muttered, almost inaudibly, "Hi, Doc."

"Well, Charles," I said, "I've read in your chart about what happened last night. I'm sorry it happened, but I'm sure glad they could revive you."

"I wish they hadn't done it," Charles said, looking me straight in the eye.

"Why?" I stammered. We had been doing everything in our power to help Charles live, and now he was telling us he wished he'd died? What was the point of our medical care if this was how he responded?

"Because if they hadn't, I wouldn't be here, like this, now," he said, sadly but matter-of-factly. His meaning was clear as he turned away from me.

Frankly, I was stunned. All my training and all my efforts had always been directed at preventing the deaths of my patients, and this honest man was telling me he didn't want that. I was perplexed and bothered, even though I understood him. Back in those days, few if any patients had advance directives, and in fact, many doctors and even some medical ethicists considered it unethical to not resuscitate whenever possible. Some still called it "killing" if a patient was not resuscitated. We were trained to do everything we could.

After recovering from this exchange, I did what a physician can always do to avoid talking—I examined Charles. But I remained troubled by his comment, so I again told him I was sorry he had the setback, and we were doing our best to get him better.

Charles smiled and simply said, "Thanks."

Later that night, at about three a.m., the phone rang. It was a nurse from the ICU. "Your patient Charles had another cardiac arrest," she said, in the caring but professional manner of an ICU nurse.

"I hope they didn't resuscitate him again," I immediately blurted.

"Well, yes, they did," the nurse responded. "It took three shocks, but they got him back."

Although I knew I couldn't do anything to help, I had to go in to see him, right then. When I entered his room he looked literally like death warmed over, eyes half-open and more pale than I had ever seen him.

As I leaned over the bed to look at him, he looked toward me and haltingly—between breaths—said, "Why … did … you … do this … to me?"

I was paralyzed for words. I struggled to understand what this gallant man was saying. Why should he accuse me—I hadn't done a thing. I wasn't even there when they did it. I didn't put the paddles to his chest and bring back unimaginably difficult breathing that both he and I knew probably would not last another full day.

"I'm sorry," is all I could say—again. He said nothing, and I left him in silence. Later that afternoon, Charles died suddenly, with no resuscitation.

But Charles's question haunted me. "Why did you do this to me?" he had asked, rhetorically. Somehow I implicitly knew he was right, in a general and more meaningful sense than my plea of personal innocence implied. Quite aside from Charles's knowledge of the pecking order in the hospital—namely that I was one of the physicians responsible for supervising the house staff who had resuscitated him—he forced me to see the larger picture of modern medicine. Charles made me understand how I and all the other physicians caring for him with our miraculous technology had put him in the condition he was in, drowning in his own lung secretions years after he would have died naturally without our help, months after his life became miserable, and now two days after he would have died without our newest technology.

We had radically changed not only *when* Charles would die but *how* he would die. Thanks to the rapid changes in technology, Charles initially did have a few more years of good life, years that Bertha never had a shot at. But in extending his life, we also extended his death, forcing him to die far more painfully and in far greater fear than Bertha had ever had to face.

Just as we changed how Charles died, we have changed how most patients die. Therefore, like it or not, we physicians are responsible for how our patients die. This is what's different now compared not just to the time of Hercules, who begged his son to help him die, but as recently as of our grandparents as well. We now die differently. And this, Charles taught me, is why physicians should change their practice habits for patients at the end of life.

Healing and Harming

I never had the chance to help save Bertha, but in helping "save" Charles's life I learned an important lesson about what it means to heal. In all the years I had known him, I had never thought to ask Charles what he wanted at the end of his life. It was not until he had endured incomprehensible suffering and been brought back from the brink of death again and again that he told me in no uncertain terms that he did not want any more of what we had to offer. But my own experience was far from unique; in fact, it was the norm. Physicians characteristically wait until there are no more nonpalliative treatment options before even discussing end-of-life care planning with their patients. For example, a study of 1,470 patients with lung or colorectal cancers found that oncologists documented end-of-life (EOL) discussions with only 27 percent of their patients, and that the discussions that patients did have were very often with health-care providers other than their oncologists, and at late stages of their illnesses—often not until the final days of their lives.[63]

The practice of doing everything possible to extend life, through scans, injections, tubes, and various medical and surgical procedures our patients endure until death is imminent, is not healing—it is pseudohealing that too often satisfies only professional needs or desires. And it fuels exactly what so many patients now fear—the extended process of dying in hospitals at the hands of physicians who are unable to let go of their traditional role as "healers."

Not only is such treatment not true healing, it can and often does harm patients. By continuing to subject patients to such invasive, uncomfortable, and painful procedures, we physicians have the potential to *harm* our patients. EOL treatment that has no reasonable chance of healing patients actually extends their suffering rather than their comfort and prevents them from experiencing their remaining life in a meaningful manner.

A case in point is that of Barney Clark, the first person to live with an artificial heart for any extended period of time. When Barney Clark lived for 112 days after his natural heart was removed, enduring four additional surgeries, endless procedures, seizures, strokes, delirium, infections, pain, and total immobility, was he not harmed?[64] I think so—inadvertently, but still harmed. Several times after having his heart removed and replaced with an artificial pump, while he was sedated, delirious, and incapacitated, he asked his physicians to let him die. Instead, they kept him alive as long as they possibly could.

Most people do not die, as Barney Clark did, tethered to a device the size of a washing machine while the entire world looks on. But many do die enduring suffering as he did—endless procedures, great pain, confusion, immobility, and compounding health problems—arising from the treatments that physicians order and not from the terminal illness itself. And they often die in noisy, brightly lit hospital rooms without privacy, sharing their rooms with absolute strangers who may themselves be dying, as a parade of health-care providers enter and leave their rooms throughout the day and night. And for many patients who are heavily sedated or comatose during their last days of life, it means they are unable to "say good-bye" and emotionally be with their loved ones at the end. It is no wonder patients would often rather die at home than in a hospital or medical institution, yet most do not get this wish because the emphasis is on healing, which all too often means treatment, compelling them to die within the medical system that treats them.

But compliance with the medical system's pull on patients to turn their disease—and death—over to the medical system in a futile effort to be healed need not be the only choice a patient can make. My own father-in-law chose a different path, one that allowed him to retain control over his remaining life once he learned the end was near. When a routine chest X-ray revealed a mass in his lung, his physicians told him it was most certainly a tumor, but he should have more tests to be sure. Although he was not having any illness symptoms other than fatigue, he knew further tests were unnecessary. Instead, he traveled, visited with his family, and generally enjoyed life for about five months. When he saw his physician again, he was once again encouraged to have more tests. But again, he refused. When his breathing became labored and he developed mental problems, he moved into a full-care nursing facility in the retirement home where his wife was also living and could visit him easily and often.

He received excellent comfort care while there, and three weeks after moving into the facility, he died. As undesired as his death may have been, by refusing further testing, in all probability my father-in-law avoided hospitalizations for surgery to remove the tumor, if not the whole lung, innumerable trips to the hospital and doctors' offices for tests, and treatments that would have included chemotherapy and probably radiation therapy, as well—leaving him far weaker and sicker than the cancer alone had left him during his final months. Like few others, my father-in-law died naturally.

I have previously raised the issue of how the concept of sanctity of life, or "living until natural death" has been hypertrophied to include unnatural means of keeping patients alive. Unfortunately, defining "natural" human life has become part of the larger "culture war" in the United States. In the Terri Schiavo case, for example, many "pro-life" adherents argued that removing Terri's feeding tube was an act of "killing," even though she was in a persistent vegetative state. Along with denying that she was in a persistent vegetative state—contrary to medical findings—they argued that she was not at the end of her natural life. This is an important cultural-religious point, because to agree that any patient being kept alive with a feeding tube is being kept alive artificially—not naturally—would be to give ground by using secular, medical criteria rather than religious criteria to define the limits of natural life. It is important, therefore, for those who advocate the sanctity of all human life to maintain the extension of life by medical technology as an extension of natural life, which is therefore subjected to "natural law" and to the sanctity-of-life principle.

In my book, *Patient-Directed Dying*,[65] I noted how Pope John Paul II argued that artificial life support was a natural process. On March 20, 2004, Pope John Paul II said that to remove the feeding tube from any patient in a persistent vegetative state would be "a serious violation of the law of God, since it is the deliberate and morally unacceptable killing of a human person."

He further stated, "I should like particularly to underline how the administration of water and food, even when provided by artificial means, always represents a natural means of preserving life, not a medical act."[66]

This quote demonstrates just how convoluted and illogical the arguments opposing PAD have become—natural deaths, like my father-in-law's are such a rarity that the artificially extended life is now viewed as the natural state!

The unshakable edict for physicians to treat disease, rather than heal the patient—a process that could require the physician to ease the patient's suffering up to and including facilitating death—leads many physicians to subject their patients to excessive treatments that intensify rather than alleviate their suffering. Just as in the movie *Wit*, where the physicians were tenaciously blinded to their patient's suffering as they stood over her, debating the progress of her cancer and their next round of treatments to destroy it, physicians often find themselves at war with a disease as their patient suffers the agonizing wounds of that war. And many doctors will avidly recommend treatments for their patients that they themselves would avoid if they were the ones dying.

This contradiction is apparent in a 2008 study of more than eight hundred physicians who had graduated from Johns Hopkins University between 1948 and 1964, regarding EOL treatment. Most of the respondents had reached their late sixties and seventies by the time of the study, so their answers were not purely hypothetical; they likely had considered the question before it was even asked of them. Asked what treatment they would accept if they'd suffered irreversible brain damage that left them unable to speak or recognize people but was not terminal, the doctors overwhelmingly said they'd decline CPR, feeding tubes, and a host of other common interventions in the event of cardiac arrest—even though they routinely recommended and used these same treatments for their patients.[67]

When true healing is no longer possible, or it is highly improbable, physicians might do better to shift to their other great duty, the relief of suffering. But relieving suffering necessitates accepting that sometimes that means helping a patient die.

In the next chapter, we turn to a discussion of medically managed dying, to better understand the role physicians can and often do play in helping patients die more gentle deaths.

CHAPTER 5
MEDICALLY MANAGED DYING

WE NOW LIVE IN a time of the medicalization of dying, or medical management of mortality, which determines how and when we die. Although most Americans would prefer to die at home, approximately 80 percent die in medical institutions, and of these, 80–90 percent die following a medical decision.[68] In short, medical treatment sets the road we take to dying. And it can be long and unpleasant. My patients Bertha and Charles suffered from the same medical problem, but how they died was determined by the treatment they did or did not get. Yet, as these cases show, there are times it becomes necessary to compromise between the desire to live and the desire to die in relative comfort by accepting potential extended suffering, a compromise the patient may well be eager to make.

Alex was one such patient. Alex was just a few months short of graduating from high school when he was diagnosed with leukemia and told he would live for no more than three or four months without treatment. He was treated with two rounds of chemotherapy and had a reasonably good result—a remission for two years before the leukemia was again out of control. After further massive doses of radiation and chemotherapy, he underwent a bone-marrow transplant. Initially the painful procedure also gave a remission, and Alex was able to live a fairly normal life for a while. But four or five months later tests showed that the leukemia had come back, and the situation was even more dire. He was kept alive for another two months with repeat visits to the hospital for multiple tests and blood transfusions and given antibiotics for one infection after another. Finally, his doctors had no more treatments to offer Alex and sent him home with hospice care. Alex died two weeks later.

Like Charles, Alex benefited from living longer with a reasonable quality of life for a while but then entered a period of terrible suffering until the end. Both Charles and Alex died in a way virtually unknown just fifty years ago—no one used to die from new health problems arising from medical treatments they'd had weeks, months, or even years before. Think about it—very few of us will escape these changes in how we die. Unless we die suddenly, as in an automobile crash or an earthquake, or from a heart attack or stroke so sudden and devastating we cannot get medical care quickly enough, we will not die naturally. We will die after medical therapy has altered our course of dying. Most of us will die under medical management.

Let's be clear about this—I'm not advocating doing away with medical treatment for otherwise fatal diseases. The benefits of modern medicine, in added months, years, and sometimes decades are enormous, and in almost all instances it would be lunacy to forego available curative treatment. The problem is not in having the treatment, although I admit that chemotherapy, bypass surgery, and the like are not akin to picnics. The problem is that there comes a point at which treatment is not doing anything to help the patient, other than extending a life that has been extinguished of any comfort, hope, or pleasure and replaced with unendurable suffering that only death can end.

The emotional highs of seeing patients gain remission from otherwise fatal illnesses are thus accompanied by the intractable anguish of deferred death. The Faustian bargain with modern medicine turns against a patient when the medical intervention or intrusion cannot be turned off. And, while it is the technology that prolongs both useful life and the end stages of dying, who, after all, is responsible for how and when medical technology is used, and the outcomes it produces? Physicians, of course.

When I was in medical school, the professor lecturing on lung cancer introduced us to the well-known aphorism, "Pneumonia is the old man's friend." A quick rush to death from pneumonia, he made clear, was preferable to the long-drawn-out suffering of the final stage of lung cancer. These days, of course, we don't allow our patients to die of pneumonia when it appears as a complication of lung cancer—we treat it, and in so doing often prolong life but also the dying process. Similarly, physicians can usually treat all the successive pneumonia-equivalent complications of most fatal diseases that would cause a quick death, not just at the beginning but throughout the course of a patient's ultimately fatal illness. The often undesirable change in the dying process begins after medical success in prolonging life, when further curing is no longer possible, and the patient arrives in the late stage of the process of dying in a condition like Alex's, or Charles's.

Ironically, much of what physicians do today, particularly in treating patients with ordinarily fatal diseases, is in fact treatment of complications of treatment. For example, antibiotics given for a lung infection can cause complications in the intestines, or result in an even worse drug-resistant infection. Radiation therapy to one area can cause damage to other nearby organs or tissues. A close friend of mine recently died of complications from treatment he needed for complications of a prior treatment that was necessary to treat complications of the original treatment of his cancer.

Physicians are fully accustomed to treating the complications of their ministrations, particularly those arising while treating otherwise fatal diseases. It's a foreseen and expected part of the unwritten contract between doctor and patient—adverse effects of interventions happen, and the physician must try to correct or alleviate any and all of them.

And they usually can do it except for one very important complication—the transforming of the patient's condition to that of incurable, prolonged dying with suffering. In this modern era of medicine, end-stage conditions are in most cases the result or complication of prior treatments, and these conditions will only get more complex in years to come. And this is why the issue of physician-assisted dying is on the front burner today.

In short, our modern way of dying often causes extended suffering at the end of life in ways we didn't face before. Instead of dying quickly at younger ages from infectious diseases such as smallpox, influenza, or pneumonia, or dying suddenly later in life from a heart attack or stroke, we are living longer lives and dying longer deaths. We now die of more gradual, long-drawn-out illnesses such as congestive heart failure, cancer, or diabetes. Today, people routinely die after prolonged dependency on artificial devices, and some live for years or decades with senility, incontinence, or prolonged unconsciousness. And, ironically, medical treatments are the reason why we are dying differently.

Of course, taking any therapy or treatment for an otherwise fatal disease is a gamble, but why must the terms of the wager be that the patient is not allowed to use the best method of limiting the loss if the gamble turns sour? Why do we put our patients in medical straightjackets at the end of life? Why won't physicians help them die more peacefully when the end has become extended suffering?

There are, in fact, two good answers to why the majority of Americans today would like to have a means of ending their dying processes quickly and peacefully. First, while we may want our lives extended as long as possible, we do not necessarily want the same of our deaths; many, if not most, people don't want to suffer endlessly once any possibility of a livable life and recovery are gone and the certainty of an agonizing death is at hand. Living without a life is not what most people want. What killed grandpa might be readily curable today, but that cure might also come at the cost of a delayed but far more undesirable death.

The second reason for the increased calls for physicians to help patients die more peacefully is that, unlike past generations, just as we have the technology to extend life, we have the medical means for peaceful dying, thereby lessening end-of-life suffering. We can do this in two ways. First, we can stop a medical treatment that is keeping someone alive, such as an artificial respirator or a feeding tube, or a patient can choose not to get a treatment such as antibiotics that would postpone dying for a while but ultimately would only prolong the dying phase. These are examples of *medically managed dying.*

Many patients get into a prolonged dying process because of their treatment, not their terminal illness. Fred didn't want to be kept alive artificially with a feeding tube inserted into his stomach. After his rounds of chemo and radiation therapy he was already in a medically managed condition, and he knew that if he went for artificial feeding he would die in a still different way than he would without further treatment.

Patients like Fred are modern examples of Heracles pleading for release, while so many physicians, like Heracles's son, refuse to treat the final complication for which they are responsible—extended suffering in the final stage of dying. We need to look at why and how dying people suffer excessively in this country, and we need to understand the denial, deception, and delusion of our medical and cultural establishments in resisting rational, compassionate, and humane methods of helping patients die peacefully. To do so, let us consider what physicians actually do to help their patients die.

The Doctor's Deception

The great irony of the claim of medical organizations and physicians who say physicians should not help their patients die is that most physicians do, in fact, help their patients die in many ways that constitute "killing" by the strict definition of the word.

Of course, they don't call it that, and I wouldn't either, as it is almost always done to relieve the suffering of dying patients. The word "kill" carries the connotation of acting without the approval of the person being killed, and while this is rarely what happens, we need to look at the many ways in which physicians routinely facilitate their patients' deaths, even while denying it. Since the dominant reason advanced against physician aid in dying is the belief that "doctors must not kill," it is important to know how some widely accepted practices of physicians are a lot closer to "killing" than is physician aid in dying. It's all in how we perceive it, and how we say it.

There are two misconceptions that allow physicians to obscure the means by which they help people die. The first is to say that if physicians are not present and directly involved with treating their patients at the time they die, the physicians are not helping them die. In order to sustain this view—a fiction, really—it becomes necessary to separate the moment of dying from the entire dying process. That is, we must isolate or uninvolve the physician and any prior medical involvement from what happens at the actual moment of dying.

As it happens, we all do this by custom. We say, the patient died "at 11:42 a.m.," or "shortly after midnight." The newspaper obituary may tell of "a long battle with cancer," but the patient "died" at a certain time on a certain day. It is true—in most cases, life ceases at a particular identifiable moment, when breathing stops and there is no pulse. But to think of death happening all at once, at a particular moment, cloaks the reality that death is the last part of a process. The dying process, as we have seen, begins with the onset of a fatal disease that, if untreated, will follow a natural course to death.

But today the dying process is fundamentally altered by modern medicine, as we have shown. When we see and describe death as happening at a clear and definable moment, rather than as a process, we fail to see, or deny, everything that physicians do that contributes to when and how the moment of death finally occurs.

A few years ago I was on a radio program debating another physician on the subject of assisted dying. After I said that physicians are very much involved in how and when their patients die, the other physician literally shouted, "Let's make this very clear—dying is not a medical event. When a patient is dying, we step back and allow them to die naturally." As we have seen, physicians do not conceptualize their unnatural treatments as producing unnatural deaths. Instead, they choose to see and describe their practices as isolated from or not part of their patients' "natural" deaths. And this is the second misconception—claiming patients die naturally.

This propensity to view death as a single, isolated event occurring at a distinct time enables us to judge the physician not by his prior artificial interventions but by what he is or is not doing at the moment of death. And it is that moment, as the Hippocratic physicians well knew, when the physician's involvement can collide with cultural principles such as sanctity of life. It is a matter of appearance—if the physician is not present and involved in a specific medical intervention at the moment of death, it would seem he is not involved in how the patient died, and therefore there is no conflict with personal or religious principles. No matter how many medical interventions the patient endures to extend life, once the physician has given up hope for a cure and stopped all treatments a day or two before the moment of imminent death, we say the patient died "naturally."

However, as we have seen, medical treatment of otherwise fatal illnesses prolongs life beyond the time of *natural* dying. Many of the objections to physician aid in dying rely on the principle that we should not help patients die but rather should allow them to die "naturally." But in fact, the whole purpose of modern medicine is to prevent natural death, whether from pneumonia, a heart attack, or cancer. None of us want to die naturally in the manner we would die without any medical or unnatural help. In fact, we can't, at least not in the United States, because almost all of us are subject to water purification, immunization, and other public health interventions that alter our lives by preventing diseases—diseases that in the developing world continue to kill people. But more importantly, because these diseases have been controlled in the developed world, and because we have access to life-saving technology, we now die differently in America. As we have seen, we now die from unnatural medical processes far more often than from direct causes of the disease itself. To better understand how this happens, let's look at some specific ways in which physicians help their patients die.

Do Not Resuscitate

The first instance of a widespread clinical practice that determined the time and mode of death of patients arose with the introduction in the 1960s of resuscitation with electrical shock to the heart, the most dramatic method of preventing death. Physicians were quick to embrace the method when they obtained the necessary equipment and developed methods of quick response to the patient whose heart had stopped. In time, resuscitation became virtually mandatory, and it was considered unethical and bad practice not to utilize it when possible.

A problem soon arose, however, when patients received multiple resuscitations—half a dozen or more in some cases. I recall one case in which the patient was resuscitated with electrical conversion seventeen times over a period of about three hours, before the physicians decided to stop. Many questioned the propriety of repeat resuscitations that predictably would not just be futile but would render harm to the patient, as happened to my patient Charles. In response to this potential problem, "do-not-resuscitate" orders, known as DNR orders, written in advance to prevent resuscitation, became increasingly common when the patient and physicians deemed further resuscitation as futile or harmful. However, some physicians and medical ethicists decried DNR orders as "killing" because it meant not bringing back to life a patient whose heart had stopped. Consequently, some physicians faced possible prosecution for failing to resuscitate a terminally ill patient in whom short-term technical success was possible.[69]

Through the decision of DNR, the physician had become involved in the time and mode of dying. The changing perception of this form of physician involvement with dying is what first engendered and later caused rejection of the use of the word "kill" to describe it. Initially, commentators focused on the isolated act, which fits the definition of "to kill," precisely because it is evident that the physician's actions or nonactions lead to the patient's death. But this connection with dying was from the start unacceptable to many physicians and medical ethicists. After the practice was redefined as "allowing the patient to die naturally," physicians could engage in DNR without the appearance of causing the deaths of their patients. Because DNR is a nonaction, the stigma of harm is removed.

Withdrawal of Life-Sustaining Therapy

Ask yourself this: When physicians destroy diseased bone marrow by treating it with chemotherapy and radiation prior to a bone-marrow transplant, is this part of natural life? Is it natural for a person to have hemodialysis once a week or more often for kidney disease? When Barney Clark died after getting "the first totally implantable heart," did he go on to die naturally? Many life-prolonging practices have been of inestimable value, but they produce a form of technology-dependent life in which natural life is maintained through machinery. By removing that machinery, however, the patient will die. Thus the perception of natural death cannot only be promoted through DNR orders but by withdrawing dramatic life-supporting therapies such as artificial ventilators, pacemakers, operations, and feeding tubes.

As the cases of Karen Ann Quinlan and Terri Schiavo showed, for as much support as there is for physician-assisted dying, the issue remains sensitive. As these early cases came to public light, there was initially volatile social reaction to the thought of removing any technological life support when a patient was unable to give voluntary consent. Throughout the mid-twentieth century, when the rapid advancement of medical science and technological innovations were impressing the medical community with the many ways in which lives could be saved and diseases or injuries managed, there was great reluctance to disconnect any potential life-saving technology. Many in the medical, legal, and religious fields considered the practice as tantamount to murder.

Thus, when physicians ordered artificial respirators or feeding tubes disconnected, many other physicians and health-care providers protested because they view such actions as violating the principles of sanctity of life and physician noninvolvement in how patients die. Of course, the physician's presence at the time the technology was removed—doing something that directly leads to the patient's death—is what made the action unacceptable. If a physician turned off an implanted pacemaker and the patient died soon after, it was hard not to believe the physician's act was responsible for the patient's death. It was the appearance of the doctor and his or her act that was troublesome, more than the act itself.

But this view began to shift in the medical community following a precedent-setting case, when the US Supreme Court established the right to refuse life support and to have it disconnected at any point. In the case of Nancy Cruzan, which we earlier touched on briefly, the justices ruled on her family's right to have her feeding tube removed, noting that "all agree that a removal of life support would cause ... death."[70] With the law on their side, many if not most physicians have now come to feel it is unethical to keep a patent alive—and suffering—through unwanted treatment. Over time, the courts and the medical profession have consequently resolved the tension between wanting to end suffering and not wanting to be perceived as delivering their patients to death, by disregarding the life-ending act of removing life-sustaining technology and viewing the dying process as simply what happens "naturally" after the treatment stops.

The Cruzan decision gave legal standing to a great semantic cover-up of physician involvement. The act of facilitating a patient's death is obscured by the way that act is described. By focusing on the underlying disease rather than the physician's act, when a physician stops treatment, the disease, rather than the doctor, kills the patient. While the health-care providers might say they "allowed" the patient to die "naturally" from the underlying disease, when a competent patient exercises her legal right to stop life-sustaining therapy, the resulting death is not viewed as the physician's doing. This semantic shift has produced a narrowing or disregarding of the physician's involvement at the time of death while deflecting the cause of death to a natural and culturally acceptable cause.

True, the disease is the underlying cause of death, but this explanation absolving the physician of involvement is sophistry based on semantic gymnastics. Let's look at a case I observed about fifteen years ago, typical of how physician-assisted dying commonly works in practice. Our patient had advanced lung disease due to cancer that had been treated for two and a half years, and he also had longstanding, severe heart disease. By then, because of heart and lung problems, the patient became unable to breathe well enough on his own to keep going, so the team of physicians hooked him up to an artificial respirator that stabilized him while the doctors tried the last remaining treatments that held any hope for reversing either of his two diseases. These efforts failed, and the doctors advised the patient and family of the situation.

The patient made a request to be disconnected from the respirator, knowing this would lead to his demise. At a meeting with his family, pastor, and two close friends, all tearfully supported him in his request. At the designated time, the doctor in charge first gave him sufficient medication to be sure he would not be aware of suffocation, and then, when all were ready, the physician disconnected him from the machine. As most often happens, once off the respirator, the patient did have some very shallow, intermittent breathing, and then gasps, and died ten minutes after the life support was withdrawn.

The doctor had a socially acceptable means of helping his patient die without it being called "killing." He could tell the family that the patient returned to his natural condition and was *allowed to die naturally*. Think about it—did the doctor's act cause the patient to die?

Now I must tell you, dear reader, I was the physician. And very clearly, I knew my act led to the patient's death. There was no escaping it. I gave the order to stop and disconnect the respirator, following which the patient died, sure as pulling the switch on an electric chair kills a convict.

Granted, I had lots of company, as there were three or four other physicians deeply involved in the patient's management, and they had all contributed to the patient's condition and concurred in the decision to disconnect the ventilator and let him die. But to say such a death is not a medical event, or that physicians were not involved in his dying, is a deception on the laity. Perhaps worse, it is a symptom of the self-delusion of physicians about their modern role in helping patients die. Actually, most physicians understand their active role in such a death, and like me they don't like doing it, but they are willing to do so at the request and for the benefit of the patient. But when physician leaders and medical experts and even justices of the US Supreme Court say the act is letting the patient die naturally, and deny the physician's role in this form of physician aid in dying, what's missing?

It's a denial of causation, pure and simple. The physician's act caused the patient to die, which, sadly, falls within the definition of "killing" used by those who oppose physician aid in dying for ideological reasons. Causation is an important legal principle. As lawyers are fond of saying, "But for this or that ... this would not have happened." Or, in this case, "But for the physician's act of disconnecting the respirator, the patient would not have died when he did."

But in this case, did I, the physician, "kill" the patient? Not in the usual sense of the word. We use a linguistic convention to sidestep the rigidity of the word "kill," for which I and most physicians are grateful. In one case in which the family asked the hospital to remove the ventilator from their daughter who had suffered irreversible brain damage, a local newspaper ran a headline, "Father Wants to Kill Daughter." Such a headline may have accurately described the consequences of disconnecting her life support, but its greater psychosocial meaning—that it was killing, and doing so was shocking and unacceptable—were powerfully conveyed in choosing to dramatize and prejudice the article with such a heading.

But language does not bend easily, and the unbending ideology that leads to the injunction "doctors must not kill" is dishonest in masking what physicians do. In fact, the most ardent of the ideological opponents of physician aid in dying still say that disconnecting a ventilator or pulling out a feeding tube to allow a terminally ill patient to die is "killing," while the great majority of people now think otherwise. We tend to lean on the circumlocution that is expressed by "allowing to die naturally," which eases our consciences but masks our direct involvement in helping patients die.

Make no mistake; if your physician responds to your request for physician aid in dying by saying, "Oh, I can't do that, doctors don't kill," more likely than not he or she says it because it is a convenient, professionally acceptable way of putting you off. But whatever the physician's purpose in saying it, such a claim is the result of a cultural-religious taboo, not actual physician practice.

Double Talk

Perhaps the most blatant professional delusion about the true nature of an act involves the so-called "double effect" of death following a high dose of a narcotic, when it is said to be given to relieve pain but given in a large enough dose that it causes death.

In 1957, a group of doctors put this question to Pope Pius XII: "Is the suppression of pain and consciousness by the use of narcotics ... permitted by religion and morality to the doctor and the patient (even at the approach of death and if one foresees that the use of narcotics will shorten life)?"

The pope replied, "If no other means exist, and if, in the given circumstances, this does not prevent the carrying out of other religious and moral duties: Yes."[71]

In this updating of an old medical principle, the pope suggested that if death is in no way intended or sought, and the intention is simply to relieve pain, the doctor is morally and religiously correct. Notice the two effects: relief of pain is intended, while death is "foreseen but unintended," as medical ethicists say.

In common medical practice, employing the "double effect" refers to administering morphine slowly and continuously, usually intravenously or beneath the skin. At any given moment in almost every major hospital in the United States, someone is dying with the help of a morphine drip. Of course, if the prime purpose is relief of pain, the dosage must be high enough to do the job. But morphine in high doses can and often does stop breathing, leading to death, and therein lies the second part of the "double effect." However, many physicians, some who are expert in using morphine, contend that doses high enough to relieve pain do not necessarily hasten or cause death. Obviously, no one can do or has done an adequate study to determine this—the lowest dose necessary to relieve pain or to cause death is different from individual to individual. But in order to relieve pain consistently, without the patient waking at intervals with screams of pain, the dose must be greater than the bare minimum necessary, which in turn can be determined only by decreasing the dosage to the point of allowing breakthrough pain. And all patients develop "tolerance" for morphine, meaning that over time higher doses become necessary. Therefore, in almost all cases, the physician uses a dose high enough to ensure blocking of all pain. Furthermore, and this is important, for morphine drips given to dying patients, the physician's order is not to give it for two or three days, or until the patient recovers, but it is open-ended, until the patient dies. As a result, the doctor's order is often for increasing the morphine dose at preset intervals, such as every six hours, to be sure the dose is high enough to suppress the pain or discomfort.

I once visited a terminally ill patient in an intensive care unit and was surprised to see no one else in the room and the bevy of machines had been removed except for a bottle dripping a clear fluid into the patient through an IV line. I decided to check the medical orders and found this: "Morphine, xx mg per hour, double the dose every four hours." Had the patient been superhuman and lived twenty-four hours, she then would have been getting sixty-four times the starting dose! As it was, she died in about eight hours. In a similar although less blatant manner, probably tens of thousands of patients die on morphine drips in our country every year. It's common practice and relieves a lot of suffering. No one knows exactly how much quicker they die from this "double effect," but every physician knows that in most cases, they would have lived longer, with more suffering, without the morphine drip. In some cases the patients would have lived a lot longer.

I am grateful for the help the morphine drip gives to many patients, and I have never found a colleague who thinks a morphine drip is wrong if the patient is suffering in the late stage of dying. But in many cases, the morphine drip is a medical wink to euthanasia, hidden by the cosmetics of professional tradition and language. It differs from the popular conception of euthanasia in two ways. The first is the old business of the physician not being there at the end. The morphine drip takes time, and family and hospital staff commonly come and go during the process. Death is gradual and appears to be of natural causes, and the doctor's absence at the time of death lets him off the hook.

The second difference that legitimizes this medical practice is based on the usually self-defined concept of the *intent* of the physician. Of course, intent is important in the law, but in assessing the intention of someone who has—let's say—shot and killed another person, there's no ambiguity of whether the alleged killer intended only to help the victim in some manner without intending to kill him. And true, doctors administer large doses of morphine to patients to relieve pain after surgery or under other circumstances, but in such cases they don't keep the patient on ever-increasing doses until death. A physician who does not *intend* his patient to die any sooner than possible will not keep that patient unconscious on morphine until the end. But, exactly because morphine is often given legitimately to relieve pain and in doses high enough to cause unconsciousness, someone observing the effect of a morphine drip for a dying patient can't tell whether the intention is to avoid death or to let it ensue.

The concept of intent in these cases is murky and an oversimplification at best—physicians themselves may be unaware of how their intention is divided between the two parts of the double effect. The ease with which physicians can say their intention was to relieve suffering and they did not intend to hasten dying hides the issue of causation, or the consequence of the physician's act. Shrouding the practice under the rubric of intent creates physician self-delusion, deception, and, ultimately, the distrust of patients.

Terminal Sedation, or Palliative Sedation

Another end-of-life medical practice, initially called *terminal sedation*, gives a similar example of physician disappearance and semantic acrobatics.[72] Doctors use this technique when, to relieve pain adequately, it is necessary to put the patient to sleep because morphine alone isn't effective in controlling it. After administering a sedative to induce a coma, the physician then withholds food and water, and the unconscious patient slowly dies through lack of liquids and nutrients. This practice is deemed ethical by the American Medical Association and legal by the US Supreme Court because a patient may exercise her constitutional right to refuse treatment (food and water), and she can give informed consent for the induced coma, which the physician gives to bring relief from symptoms, not with "intent to kill." And, of course, since the patient usually dies days after the procedure is begun, the physician is not present at the end, and the patient is said to have "died naturally, of her disease." Of course it is not natural to die of dehydration, which is what happens with this procedure.

Unfortunately, almost no patient who receives continuous sedation is mentally alert enough to give informed consent prior to starting the treatment, which is why the procedure was initially called "*terminal* sedation," reflecting the result of using it.[73] But even in the rare cases in which the patient is alert enough to give informed consent, the procedure is presented as a means of relieving pain, not ending life. Thus, this practice could be abused much more easily than physician aid in dying, which not only requires consent of the patient but is done *by the patient*, not the physicians. Terminal/palliative sedation is a far greater risk than is physician-assisted dying for vulnerable patients who do not know how to discuss end-of-life options with physicians, and who have no advocate monitoring treatment decisions for them.

Because the name "terminal" sedation indicated its purpose in sedating to death, physicians distanced themselves from both the term and the practice. One response to this public awareness was to change how the procedure was framed by calling it "*palliative* sedation," rather than terminal.[74] Thus the procedure is now presented as helping to relieve suffering, not as leading to death.

Clearly, if a patient is sedated only to relieve symptoms while hydration and nourishment are administered, it does not lead to death, as sedation alone does not kill unless grossly over-administered. As with the morphine drip, there can be a gray zone within which the ultimate effect of the sedation is difficult to judge and gives physicians a cover to use "palliative sedation" to help a patient die. In both these procedures, as well as physician aid in dying, physicians do intend to relieve suffering, but when a patient is sedated while hydration is withheld, the latter act leads to death and should be so acknowledged. Palliative sedation is now viewed as a combination of the "double effect" (anesthesia to relieve pain or suffering) and withdrawal of life-supporting treatment (nourishment and fluids), both of which are legal and generally accepted as ethical.[75]

This semantic shuffle helps many physicians and medical ethicists who do not approve of any form of overt physician aid in dying to cling to the deception that with morphine drips and palliative sedation, physicians are not involved in helping their patients die, which helps them justify the practice as conforming to their ethics. But it is specious to say that in these procedures there is no intent of helping the patient die; the doctors know that withholding fluids and nutrition invariably leads to death and that excessive morphine suppresses respiration. And such deaths are anything but natural; they constitute slow euthanasia—deliberately killing another person to end his or her suffering.[76] Moral judgment based on appearance at the time of physicians' involvement in helping patients die is medically and ethically problematic, for it denies moral responsibility for what has gone before it.[77]

What is going on here is, I believe, a desire to maintain traditional practices that incidentally allow physicians to help their patients die while banning practices that cannot be hidden under semantic posturing and seem overtly contrary to the rigid "doctors must not kill" dictum. To this end, opponents of physician aid in dying use what they call an ethical distinction between "allowing to die" and "killing." But as we've seen, they base this distinction not on actual practice but on appearance, by ignoring what happens when physicians withdraw artificial respirators or use morphine drips and other procedures in end-of-life treatment.

One physician-ethicist, an ardent opponent of physician aid in dying, says physicians may foresee and desire that their patients may die quickly from a medical act without intending that they die. In an argument that strangely conforms to the logic of Pope Pius XII, the physician explained his position by presenting a hypothetical case of a doctor withdrawing life support from a patient: "Mrs. Brown's physician can hope for her quick death; expect it; even pray for it. But this does not mean that her physician has committed herself to bringing about Mrs. Brown's death as the condition that fulfills her intention. Desire and belief are not intention."[78]

In other words, the physician expects her act will cause death, hopes for it, and even prays for it, but can turn around and say she doesn't intend it? This twisted logic is a gross self-delusion if the physician truly believes it, although I doubt many do. But it is an extreme example of how aid-in-dying opponents attempt to allow some practices but ban others that are too obvious for even this sort of sophistry.

The physician crosses the line, opponents say, if and when he accedes to the patient's request to die, by any method. Yes, it is clear, if a patient in a hospital pleads with her doctor to, "Please give me something to let me die and escape this suffering," it's hard for the physician to fool himself into thinking that the medication, even if administered as a conventional morphine drip, is not intended to cause death. This is why the patient who asks directly for help in dying will almost never get it. *The request itself makes what is happening too obvious.* On the other hand, if the plea is modified to be indirect and nonspecific, such as, "Doctor, I'm suffering so much, I can't bear it; can't you help me even if it sedates me?" the physician may well supply the necessary means. And of course, physician aid in dying in Washington and Oregon crosses the line for opponents because the patient asks for it. In addition to the direct request from the patient, by codifying the practice, those who act openly under the umbrella of the law explicitly cross the ideological line.

But while we're massaging semantics, an interesting and important fact makes the physician's intent to cause death *less certain* when participating in physician aid in dying than when disconnecting life support or using palliative sedation. When a physician disconnects a patient from a respirator on which the patient is dependent to stay alive, or gives a patient continuous sedation while stopping nutrition and hydration, the probability of the patient dying as a result of the act approaches 100 percent. Yet, under the laws of Washington and Oregon, when a physician writes a prescription for life-ending medication for a dying patient, the probability that the physician's act will lead to the death of the patient is less than 65 percent. This lower rate of mortality is because more than a third of patients who get the medication under the law never take it or die first from progression of their diseases. So, ironically, a physician acting under a physician aid in dying law is *less* likely to cause his patient to die than a physician whose act "allows the patient to die naturally."

But then, the true reason for the alleged distinction between "killing" and "allowing to die" regarding these common end-of-life practices is ideological. From Hippocrates to the hypocrisy of the "double effect," physicians have, by strict definition, killed their patients to relieve their suffering, even if the word "kill" is misleading and entirely unsuited to the act. The confounding professional difference between physician aid in dying and the ideologically justified methods of helping patients die through medically managed dying is how these practices are presented to the public. And maintaining the myth of the difference between "killing" and "allowing to die" requires doctors and other health professionals to weave a web of remote probabilities and unspoken secondary intentions—the surest way of screening themselves and their patients from the truth. The self-deluding semantic umbrellas under which doctors can and do help their patients die creates professional, legal, and social distortion of medical practices, and in the process deceives the public.

Does this mean those physicians who resist openly engaging in physician-assisted dying are any more (or less) ethical than those who do? What leads physicians to oppose a practice they actually engage in, beyond the cognitive dissonance necessary to placate a troubling conscience? Those who oppose the practice or shroud it in linguistic finery are not insensitive to suffering. They are conforming to professional imperatives that their professional culture dictates and are shaped by their particular specializations, which determine and limit the treatment strategies they pursue.

In the next chapter, we explore these "professional imperatives" in more detail and consider the role that changes in the medical system, including the increased use of hospice care and changing health-insurance coverage, now plays in changing how and when we die.

CHAPTER 6
PROFESSIONAL IMPERATIVES

"**I** DON'T DO THAT," is usually the specialist's response when a patient asks for help with dying. Consider for a moment Fred's physician, the patient in chapter 3 who asked for help with dying when his cancer could no longer be controlled. Fred said to his doctor, "Well, I expect to get better, and I'm hoping for a cure. But I know that with a disease like this, sooner or later it will get the better of me. When that happens, and a cure is no longer possible, at the end, Doctor, will you help me die peacefully?"

"You've come to me to help you live, not to die," said the oncologist, who then said good-bye and left the room. Why did the oncologist refuse to talk about the possibility of physician aid in dying if or when the treatment failed? And when the end did come, why did the oncologist refuse to consider physician aid in dying and say, "There is nothing more we can do for you."

The physician was not misleading Fred; he actually believed there was nothing more he could do. He was in denial of the options available to the dying and of his ability to help. The underlying reasons for this sort of denial are complex and often arise from physicians' training.

Fred's physician was an oncologist, and as such he did what he was trained to do—he treated him with chemotherapy. When the first chemotherapy drug didn't work any longer, he was ready to treat him with another one. And then another. It was his job to know what worked, and to do his best to make it work for his patient's benefit. And he did a good job doing what he knew how to do—but that wasn't the problem at the end. As an oncologist, he was trained to treat cancer. What the oncologist refused to do was recognize and help with the multitude of other end-of-life conditions that his cancer treatments had helped create for Fred. In a real sense, his treatment led to untreatable complications, and at the end these complications caused Fred far more suffering than did the cancer alone.

Yet if the law permits physicians to withdraw treatment, as well as to provide palliative treatment that might hasten death, why did Fred's physician—all of his physicians for that matter—resist helping him under the law?

From his first visit with Fred, the oncologist was displaying a potent characteristic of specialists—a positive desire and drive to do what he was trained to do. Doing what he or she is trained to do is the easiest thing for a physician to do—it's the physician's comfort zone. Other approaches are not only more difficult but would likely prevent the physician from doing what comes naturally after years of education and practice.

This "function-lust," or the love of performing a function, is common to all professions, artisans, and craftsperson.[79] The baker wants to bake and the lawyer wants to litigate, and when given the opportunity each will drive headstrong to do what he or she does best, often to the exclusion of other ways of preparing food, resolving a conflict, or helping a patient. Function-lust creates a necessity for physicians to use a technique or skill in order to maintain their skills, their purpose, and their reputations. Indeed, were they not to do what they were trained to do, these professionals would risk being faulted not only for inaction but for transgressing into territory where they lack expertise—in other words, presuming an expertise for which they may have no training.

Furthermore, for an oncologist (or any specialist, for that matter), it is far worse to miss the opportunity for a treatment success than to have a treatment fail. The specialist who doesn't "do everything possible" to cure the patient risks the displeasure of colleagues who observe that the physician has made less than an "all-out" effort, which in turn could create a risk of diminishing referrals. To not succeed at what one is uniquely qualified to do is professionally and personally unacceptable. A surgeon will most likely pick up his knife if an operation holds even a small chance of success for a dying patient. A treatment failure, on the other hand, only demonstrates the imperfect nature of therapy and the variability of individual response to it. A treatment failure is seldom seen as a failure of the physician unless he or she hasn't done it properly.

Just as in warfare, few generals practice the reasonable retreat; it is far better to go into battle and lose honorably than to not do battle at all. And so it is with physicians in the "frontlines" of a battle against death and disease. Few will retreat when there is still the opportunity to advance and attack—which is done by treating the patient to the best of the physician's ability.

Nowhere is this tunnel-vision principle of not straying from the job better demonstrated than in dealing with medical specialists. Theoretically, and probably in reality as well, the nonspecialist, or generalist, is best suited by temperament and practice habits to direct a patient's overall care, including a discussion of all options. But a patient such as Fred is usually fated to deal with several specialists—sometimes a half dozen or more—all of whom focus on their particular function, while the generalist fades into the background, ill-equipped to challenge the expertise of specialists.

This changing face of medicine and the US medical system has had profound implications for all areas of health care, but its impact has perhaps been most notable in end-of-life care.

"Decisions about continuation of treatment are influenced by the enthusiasm of the doctors who propose them," Sherwin Nuland, a surgeon, explains. "Commonly, the most accomplished of the specialists are also the most convinced and unyielding believers in biomedicine's ability to overcome the challenge presented by a pathological process close to claiming its victim."[80] The rapidly advancing successes of science and technology to control and manage nature have infused medical specialists with a certainty that nature can be controlled, and that disease can consequently be controlled, if not conquered.

In the context of biomedicine, assisted dying is so outside the conventional practice of medicine that for many physicians it falls under the umbrella of alternative or rogue therapies—something few physicians are willing to contemplate. For Fred's oncologist to do what he wanted to do, which was to do everything in his power to prolong Fred's life, he could not afford to spend time on alternatives, much less one that might shorten the duration of his job. For him it was a professional imperative *not* to discuss—much less engage in—aid in dying as an end-of-life option. To do so would constitute a step back in time on the continuum of medical knowledge, to relinquish the power of biomedicine in favor of a simple "natural remedy."

Thus, to achieve his goals, the specialist strives to eliminate or at least defer discussion of alternative courses of treatment or anything that might diminish the patient's compliance with the recommended treatment.

The Power of Hope

Function-lust is not the only professional imperative that influences physician behavior. It would be remiss not to mention the financial incentives constantly at work under our medical system. Most of the specialists I know are fine, dedicated people who would not knowingly and purposely alter a patient's treatment for financial gain. On the other hand, the most dedicated physicians are influenced, whether consciously or unconsciously, by financial incentives. If coronary bypass surgery, or CT scans, or even many types of chemotherapy did not reimburse physicians at such a high level as is the case in our "get paid for everything you do" medical system, it is probable far fewer of these treatments would be recommended to dying patients.

Given the lucrative nature of ordering such procedures for patients, particularly when an insurance company or Medicare rather than the patient will pay for a procedure, even the most well-meaning and ethical of physicians may easily find themselves routinely ordering such tests. After all, they reason, doing so has the potential to help the patient and certainly cannot harm him or her. But the harm, as we have seen, may not necessarily come from any one test or surgical procedure but from the cumulative nature of continually subjecting the suffering patient to more and more invasive procedures that over time become a form of tender-loving torture.

If physicians are reluctant to help their patients die because they view it as outside their job description, they have failed their patient. But doctors do not intend to fail their patients; as we have seen, quite to the contrary, they want more than anything to succeed. It is the physician's tenacity to succeed in the face of certain death that fuels their efforts to keep patients alive beyond their natural demise.

But there is another factor shaping physician resistance to assisted death that is far more subtle than anything we've discussed thus far. And that is the belief that the physician must never let the patient give up hope.

The refusal to consider assisted dying if or when treatment is no longer effective is the flipside of hope, and is founded on our culture's deep belief in the "power of positive thinking." Hope has been the eternal maidservant of the healer. It may be an open question of whether hope itself is efficacious in affecting the course of a fatal disease, but throughout history no healer of any stripe has succeeded in the minds of his or her patients and observers without instilling hope in the treatment being offered or given. Conversely, the absence of hope will surely undermine any healer, be he an ancient priest-healer or a modern medical specialist. To the modern physician, it too often seems self-evident that to discuss options for dying is to chip away at the healer's best friend—hope. Indeed, to the physician dependent upon the elixir of hope, the pursuit of death is an audacious rejection of hope. In its place, the physician offers her own form of hope, however remote, through treatment options.

As any physician knows, the patient's confidence in the treatment and hope for its success are critical to the undertaking. In other words, the physician must be an arch-advocate for what he is proposing, and this seems fair enough—someone must forcefully advocate for what is generally considered the best treatment for an otherwise fatal disease, without discussing what to do if it doesn't turn out well. All physicians, but specialists in particular, want patients who are willing to go all the way—physicians want every chance to succeed. After all, patients and peers alike are judging doctors by how they succeed with their therapies, not by how they help their patients die.

Fred's physician refused his request for help with dying—not because he thought Fred *would* beat his cancer but because to agree to the request would be to concede there was no hope for total success for Fred, and without hope, both Fred and the physician had failed. At that point, in the physician's view the cancer would no longer be what was killing Fred; it would be the decision to give up hope that was going to kill him. And while the oncologist might not be able to instill any more hope in Fred, he was not about to renounce it himself. His success depended upon remaining as optimistic as possible for as long as possible.

This faith in optimism has long played a central role in American culture, from the founding of the nation to the emergence and perpetuation of "the American Dream." This optimism has instilled the national character with a spirit that has enabled it to overcome, at different times in our history, great adversity, including the shackles of slavery, the economic collapse of the Great

Depression, civil and world wars, and desperate poverty. The idea that an elusive power resides in the universe that can reverse our course through sheer faith has provided immense comfort to the suffering. This view has taken a multitude of forms, from Norman Vincent Peale's Depression-era *Power of Positive Thinking*, to the present glut of self-help books, inspirational leaders, and personal coaches advocating visualization, affirmations, and unshakable faith that all will be well through hope alone.

This thinking can even go so far as to advise that all health problems can be conquered through optimism alone. For example, in the phenomenally popular best seller *The Secret*, author Rhonda Byrne compiled quotations from writers and philosophers concerning the "power" of optimism to suggest that there exists a scientific principle that compels good things to happen to people who think good thoughts. Extending these ideas into the realm of health and illness, she advises, "It is as easy to heal a pimple as a disease. The process is identical, the difference is in our minds … nothing is incurable. At some point in time, every so-called incurable disease has been cured. In my mind, and in the world I create, 'incurable' does not exist. There is plenty of room for you in this world … it is the world where 'miracles' are everyday occurrences."[81]

Of course, not everyone believes healing cancer is as easy as healing a pimple. But the book sold millions of copies because it resonated with the deeply held view in our culture that we can overcome even the greatest adversity by harnessing our thoughts toward magnificent ends.

There is no question that hope and optimism can improve patients' sense of well-being. The issue here is not whether hope is desirable for most patients, which it is, but whether *false* hope can cause excess suffering. There does come a time in every life when no amount of optimism and hope can prevent our deaths; we all die. And I have seen too many patients and their families fight desperately to live, believing as long as they possibly could that they would beat their disease, only to finally reach a point when optimism could no longer conceal the cruel truth—they were going to die. And when that point is reached, the best role for hope and optimism is for the patient and his or her family to hope for the kindest death possible.

But to the physician who wants the patient to maintain hope for a longer life, false hope might snuff out the one last chance for a gentle death. For in the medical setting it is the physician who is in control, and the physician who will decide whether or not the patient will have help in dying. And that is not patient-centered medicine, it is physician-centered medicine.

Palliative Care

But what happens when the patient challenges the physician to relinquish control in order to let the patient die, or even to direct the dying process toward aid in dying? To ease the tension between the patient's quest for relief from suffering and the physician's quest for control over patient care, and to justify not helping their patients die, many physicians have a fallback. And that fallback is the myth that hospice care alone will provide the patient with what he or she truly wants—to die in peace and free of suffering. Hospice care is, in my opinion, one of the great advances of the last forty years—it has provided great relief of suffering for many patients. The issue is not whether it is effective, which it so often is, but whether hospice care is *always* sufficient to relieve end-of-life suffering.

Some physicians actively oppose physician aid in dying because they say comfort care, also known as palliative care or optimal medical treatment, is sufficient to eliminate or control symptoms at the end of life. Many hospitals now have "palliative care" units just for this purpose, as well as for symptom control of patients who are not dying. But where comfort or palliative care is most commonly practiced is in hospices, where providing comfort to patients at the end of life is the primary goal.

Hospices have a long history dating back to the eleventh century during the early era of the Crusades. While heretics might not have fared well in the hands of these religious Crusaders, the terminally ill fared better. Christians suffering from incurable diseases were housed in places set aside for the care of the dying. In the centuries that followed, various forms of this "hospice" treatment were provided throughout Europe. But it wasn't until the 1980s that the modern hospice movement, first started in England, became popular in the United States when AIDS began afflicting hundreds of thousands of people who were in need of end-of-life care. By the mid-1990s, hospice care was well established, and virtually all hospitals in the United States are now affiliated with some form of hospice program, and the service— which may require twenty-four-hour home care—is now covered by Medicare and most insurance plans. Because hospice care has been so successful, however, many physicians now believe it is sufficient for the terminally ill and consequently makes physician-assisted dying unnecessary.

Not only do many physicians consider the success of hospices a justification for not legalizing physician-assisted dying, those who provide hospice and palliative care as their specialty also tend to resist PAD for this same reason. As a result, many opponents of PAD argue that if those who specialize in helping people die in comfort see no need for helping people die, it must not be necessary. But this reasoning provides only a circular argument, just as heart surgeons are the ones most in favor of surgery for heart ailments, and cardiologists tend to be more in favor of angioplasties than surgeries. The fact that those who provide comfort end-of-life care believe the care they provide is sufficient for all patients should come as no surprise. It is yet another professional imperative that they have faith in what they do.

Unfortunately, specialists in palliative care are as subject to function-lust as any other type of specialist. As one specialist in end-of-life palliative care defined her job: "good palliative medicine neither prolongs nor shortens life ... to help a patient die would change my reality forever. It would alter the way doctors, nurses, and other caregivers see each other and see patients. I would never see a patient again without asking myself a series of questions, such as: 'At some arbitrary time, will the family say, "Now, this is it?"' Or is it up to the physician to decide when the quality of life ends?"[82]

In other words, she was saying she doesn't want to change her job or how she perceives her role in end-of-life care.

Another palliative-care expert physician noted that none of her colleagues would consider physician aid in dying because it is not what they do: "All of the physicians are 'opting out' of DWD [death with dignity]. This is being done not necessarily because they are philosophically opposed to it; rather, these physicians want to be clear with patients who are going through the DWD process that they will not be writing the prescription and that their only aim is to relieve pain and suffering, clarify the goals of care and optimize quality of life."[83]

Oh, if only the "good palliative care is sufficient" argument were true! If it were, we would all die with less suffering. Unfortunately, although hospice care does indeed provide invaluable end-of-life care, facts seriously rebut the claim that this care is sufficient for every patient. A recent report summed up the state of the issue in its title: "Cancer Doctors Still Not Great with Patients' Pain."[84] The pain of dying can be beyond control, regardless of the care and resources provided to the patient. While palliative and hospice care can control symptoms and allow peaceful dying for the majority of dying patients, it is not unusual for hospice patients to report pain or shortness of breath during the last week of life as being severe or intolerable.

It may be true that following weeks or even months of palliative care, in which the patient's comfort has been well managed, one week of suffering may not seem extreme to some physicians. Yet if that last week of pain and suffering were cruelly inflicted upon a person without a medical problem—in other words, if a person were intentionally tortured to death—we would view that suffering quite differently. If a killer slowly suffocated his victim for as long as a week, or inflicted excruciating pain for seven or more days before ultimately killing his victim, any one of us would find such suffering heinous, a horrific form of torture that no one should endure. One week of suffering horribly will be experienced as a form of unnecessary suffering regardless of its cause; while there may be greater fear at the hands of a killer, when those final days of extreme suffering can be brought to a swift end but that end is denied, the one who suffers may not distinguish one form of suffering from another. It can indeed be torture to die, especially when that death takes days.

In addition to pain, many patients suffer in other ways that may not be painful but can be extremely disturbing and often uncontrollable, such as shortness of breath, choking, vomiting, diarrhea, extreme weakness and fatigue, loss of bowel or bladder control, and delirium. Few people understand how distressing is the extreme fatigue many patients dying of cancer have. In these cases, palliative care is less effective.

And, unfortunately, palliative treatment often has unwanted side effects that over and above all else can make dying unbearable. These side effects include severe constipation due to morphine and sedation caused by many of the drugs used to control symptoms. Although enough medication can put any patient to sleep, thereby relieving symptoms, many patients do not want to be "drugged" for the last days or weeks of their lives. Also, while relieving pain is an excellent way to help a patient's feeling of well-being, intensive palliative care does not help with the more existential aspects of dying, such as the desire of many dying patients to be in control of their final days. They may not want to be—or even feel as if they are—a burden on others, or suffer the indignities of soiling the bed, communicating with family and friends under the influence of drugs and delirium, and otherwise being left in a state of infantile dependence.

Ideological opponents of physician aid in dying commonly belittle these desires as just a desire for control, but they are extremely important to many dying patients. Exactly what constitutes intolerable suffering is best defined by the patient and may occur in ways not noticed or understood by physicians, whose roles, as we have seen, are often limited by their training and the professional culture in which they function.

Yet even the leading hospice group, the National Hospice and Palliative Care Organization (NHPCO), which may not consider legalized physician-assisted dying necessary, does recognize the limitation of palliative care: "Suffering can occur even when physical symptoms are well controlled. As with any other type of suffering, NHPCO believes that hospice and palliative-care professionals have an ethical obligation to respond to existential suffering using the knowledge, tools, and expertise of the interdisciplinary team."[85]

The claim that physician aid in dying is not necessary because good comfort care is sufficient rings loudly false when one considers the patient who understands that good palliative care may well lead to a peaceful death at the end with minimal or no suffering, but wishes to have options available if that care cannot provide a relief from suffering. For these patients, their desire to terminate the dying process while still able to interact with family and friends—and not linger for weeks while heavily sedated and dependent on others for basic personal needs—is a legitimate concern and one that, in my view, ought be considered as a basic human right.

Think about it for a few seconds. Any physician knows well the potential suffering possible during the last days or weeks of life, despite the best efforts of comfort care, as we mentioned in chapter 4.[86] Physicians, just like their patients, want control over their final days; they want to die with dignity. And many of them do; given their access to the resources necessary to do so—medications, technology, sympathetic fellow physicians— many physicians who oppose legalized PAD know the issue won't affect them. They are assured of aid in dying should it become necessary. Why, then, are their patients so commonly denied this same assistance?

Even if both methods—comfort care and physician aid in dying—are effective in facilitating the best possible end-of-life care, why should one method exclude the other? No physician would argue that legalized PAD would put the hospice industry out of business—if anything, physicians who support PAD are strong supporters of hospice care because they know it may provide the very care their patients seek, and that it may well make PAD unnecessary. Yet at the same time, they also know that it may not be enough.

But those who argue that palliative care renders physician aid in dying unnecessary use the premise that since the one option often works, the other option should never be considered. Such a leap requires more than faith in the efficacy of palliative care—it reflects some further, unstated objection to physician aid in dying. Could it be a mere professional imperative that influences their thinking, a belief that to acknowledge the limitations of their care means they have failed? Could it be a concern that given the fact that they are the end-of-life caregivers, legalized PAD might tarnish their reputations, casting a shadow upon their roles and marking them as potential angels of death, rather than comfort providers? Whatever the reasons that many palliative care physicians resist legalized PAD, one thing is certain: the explicit claim that PAD is unnecessary because their work is so efficacious—which it clearly is in many if not most cases—is a specious one. Even the best palliative care is sometimes not enough to spare the dying unnecessary suffering, suffering we have the technological means to end swiftly, gently, and humanely.

Why Physicians Don't Help Their Patients Die

Why, then, should palliative care experts control how we die, rather than put control in the hands of the patients themselves? The physician who says palliative care is sufficient for *all* dying patients is using a false cover—he or she just doesn't want to use physician aid in dying, whether the reason for resisting it is professional, social, or religious. The issue is not whether palliative care can control symptoms but who decides how and when the patient should die. Must physicians control everything about how and when a patient dies? This all-too-prevalent attitude does not represent patient-centered medicine—it is physician-centered medicine.

There is one other reason physicians have been resistant to embrace legalized PAD, and it concerns the issue of confidentiality. Whether done secretly and outside the law or legally under the laws of Oregon, Washington, or Montana, in most cases physicians must take confidentiality measures so their act does not become known within the profession or among the general public.

The need for confidentiality arises because of the potentially damaging effect when opponents of PAD publicize or "out" a physician for engaging in it, just as in cases of physicians performing lawful abortions who find themselves picketed, harassed, and even killed in rare cases. No physician wants to have to deal with hostile publicity, replete with the usual charges of "murder" or "killing." There is also the need to maintain confidentiality for the patient's family, who for many reasons usually do not want the matter publicized. The fear of adverse publicity can be so great that it inhibits many physicians from helping their patients die, even when they are otherwise willing to do so.

The confidentiality issue is even more pressing in communities that have higher numbers of PAD opponents. I well remember a dying patient who wanted to use the Oregon Death with Dignity Law to obtain peaceful dying. He had an aggressive cancer, and shortly after it was first diagnosed and he had begun treatment, he asked his longtime family physician to help him under the law if and when he became terminally ill and his death was near. The doctor agreed, and as it happened, the treatment was of limited help, the cancer spread, and the patient was told by several specialists he had only a few more months to live. So the patient returned to his family doctor and asked for the help he had been promised.

But the doctor hesitated and said, "I want you to think about this and come back in a week and we'll talk about it then."

A week later the patient returned, confident his doctor would follow through with his promise now that the patient had shown he had indeed thought the matter over and knew what he was doing.

But to his surprise, his doctor told him, "I'm sorry, I can't help you. I just can't do it."

I had known the doctor professionally, and at the patient's request, I phoned him to ask why he had refused to help his dying patient.

"Look," he confided in me, "I don't mind helping patients die, but I don't want to do it under the law."

I was taken aback by his answer and asked, "Why not? If you want to help him, why not use the law?"

"You just don't understand the private practice of medicine," he said. "All my colleagues have told me not to do it, that it wouldn't be good for our clinic. And my wife came home from church recently and told me all the women at her church had told her I shouldn't be doing it. That was the last straw—there is just no way I can do it."

The irony, of course, is that this physician and many like him support in principle the practice of helping terminally ill patients die in order to lessen their suffering. And, in fact, they sometimes do it. But when they do, they do it privately, as they have for years. But they don't want it known in the community or in the profession for fear of being branded a murderer. And assisting the dying under the law might mean others would learn about it, defeating the effort to assist the dying discreetly and privately.

This desire by physicians to assist their patients privately and free of the judgmental eyes of a hostile public that opposes PAD is certainly understandable. But it is yet another form of physician-centered medicine, where the patient receives the treatment that best suits the needs of the physician, not the patient.

The ramifications of physician-centered medicine are reflected not just in the care a patient receives but in patients' understanding just what care is possible. Many hospice caregivers are like physicians in that they do not view their professional duty to be helping patients die; they view their role as providing comfort. Consequently, even in states such as Washington or Oregon, where physician aid in dying is legal, many hospice patients do not receive information about this option and do not have full access to it.[87] In order to ensure patients have the best care available to them at the ends of their lives, and to be able to make informed decisions about that care, legalizing PAD is not only necessary, it requires a shift in consciousness on the part of physicians and end-of-life caregivers. The professional imperatives of these skilled and caring caregivers must be challenged to provide room for PAD in the cognitive, social, and emotional realms in which end-of-life caregivers and physicians operate.

I believe physicians like the one who refused to help Fred shorten his days of suffering are more than just mistaken in their reasons for denying help. Although I sympathize with physicians who refuse to openly help their patients die because they fear social or professional criticism or even ostracism, I believe physicians as a whole are in many respects delusional about the effects of some of the things they do for end-of-life care and what they think they shouldn't do. Like those in other professions, they tend to act in their own self-interest. The doctors' delusion will add ever more to our suffering until they learn to better serve their patients, not themselves. But to get there, we must create a social climate that makes this shift in thinking possible.

In the next chapter I reflect on this changing social climate and explore the laws and public debates that shape the practice and perspectives of physician-assisted dying.

Chapter 7
Legal and Political Issues

WHEN FRED ASKED HIS doctor to help him die and his doctor refused, it could be understandable if doing so were a crime. But Fred and his doctor were in Oregon, a state that since 1994 has allowed physicians to prescribe a lethal dose of medication for their terminally ill patients to take if and when the patients choose to do so. But the law itself has proven insufficient for many patients, given the continuing resistance of physicians to put it into practice. And of those who do ask their physicians for a prescription to end their suffering, only about one in six get it.[88] Undoubtedly, one of the reasons there is such a low rate of physician compliance is because many of those patients who request the medication don't qualify under the terms of the law; to qualify, a patient must be terminally ill with fewer than six months to live, be a resident of the state, and be of sound mind and capable of making a rational decision to die. Yet even when patients do meet these criteria, many physicians are still resistant to openly assist their patients to die.

Physicians point to the risk of legal trouble if they help a patient die, given that PAD is legal in only three states (Oregon, Washington, and Montana). And nothing will inhibit a doctor more quickly and thoroughly than the threat of being hauled before a judge or a medical-review committee. One physician in Washington State told me he would never act to help a patient die under the law because he was certain he would be harassed and prosecuted by the state for doing so.

Nevertheless, and in fairness to physicians, some do knowingly help their patients die if and when not dying means prolonged suffering. But except for Oregon, Washington, and Montana (and possibly Hawaii*), physicians who give aid in dying do so illegally and in secrecy, as we have discussed in chapter 5.

Even though practiced to some extent in the majority of states where it remains illegal, indictment for illegally engaging in PAD is exceedingly rare. Even Dr. Kevorkian—who wanted publicity for what he did—was acquitted in trials three times, while the fourth was declared a mistrial. Only when the CBS television show *60 Minutes* showed Dr. Kevorkian ending a patient's life—not by PAD but by euthanasia, which is to say injecting the non-terminally ill patient with lethal drugs rather than the patient self-injecting—was he convicted of second-degree homicide. Thus, despite their fears of legal or professional troubles arising from engaging in PAD, the reality for physicians is that the risks of such trouble are rare. Indeed, were it not for this awareness, physicians would not continue to practice it, as many routinely do.

As we've seen, physicians are unwilling to help patients die for a myriad of reasons. Their objections arise not from opposition to relief of suffering but from an aversion to relieve suffering by actively intervening to bring the dying process to a quicker end. Some of this aversion may be associated with a sense of guilt, but ultimately, the reasons for denying patients legal help in dying are usually social or professional imperatives or inhibitions, or religious or cultural prohibitions against ending life by any means. And often it's some of both.

---

* Although there is no specific death-with-dignity law in Hawaii, a unique law dating to 1909 provides terminally ill patients with considerable freedom to control their own deaths, leaving the issue of physician-assisted death unclear and open to interpretation at present.

The case of Terri Schiavo, discussed in chapter 1, reflects this dual motivation to resist assisted dying. The bitterness between the two sides in this case was nothing short of excruciating—a husband who wanted his irreversibly brain-damaged wife disconnected from life support, and parents who wanted their daughter to live, however damaged—and testifies to the far-reaching political, legal, and cultural ramifications that are possible in conflicts over how we die. The culture war was in full swing as the Schiavo case played itself out in the public arena, and physician aid in dying has become an ever-larger part of this cultural war. And one powerful symbol of this conflict, one that bears directly on sentiments related to assisted dying, is the issue of abortion.

The ideological opposition to abortion has focused on physicians, abortion clinics, and hospitals. For decades in this country, ideologically driven and well-organized protests have prevented physicians and clinics from providing this legal medical service for women. Protests have been organized outside the offices and clinics of physicians and caregivers who practice abortion, "shame" tactics are used to "expose" physicians who practice abortions—and sometimes even their patients who have them— by videotaping them or writing blogs or articles that are posted on the Internet. Physicians who provide abortions are blacklisted, and in some cases shot at, injured, or even killed. These aggressive and violent tactics have created a culture of secrecy around a legal practice. Other tactics that have suppressed women's right to abortion have included cutting off access to legal abortions through institutional restrictions, such as Catholic hospitals and clinics banning providers from providing abortions and birth control, or laws that block public funding of institutions or agencies that provide or advise women of their right to abortion. Similarly, birth control medication has now become restricted for increasing numbers of patients by the rising practice of insurers refusing coverage on the ostensible grounds of ideological opposition.

These tactics that have proven successful in preventing women from gaining access to legal abortion are being replicated in many ways throughout Washington and Oregon, as patients seek access to legalized physician-assisted dying. In areas where the only hospital is Catholic-run, and particularly where most or all of the physicians are employed by a Catholic health-care group (as is the case in some areas), many or most physicians are banned from participating in physician aid in dying. Thus, in some areas, a minority ideological view prevents access for the majority.

The problem is now becoming more widespread with the trend toward financially based mergers of Catholic and secular hospitals, where even in Washington and Oregon legalized PAD can become thwarted by organizational imperatives. When a secular hospital merges with a Catholic one, the Catholic hospital will inevitably insist that any merger include a prohibition of physician aid in dying on its premises or by its physicians, meaning the newly merged hospitals will follow the Catholic directives regardless of the secular hospital's prior policy. Because the laws in Washington and Oregon have an opt-out provision that permits individual institutions from participating in PAD, the law cannot ensure that patients will have access to PAD just because it is legal.

This allowance to opt out of participation in physician aid in dying is a necessary and desirable expression of constitutionally guaranteed free expression of religion. But given the disproportionate number of Catholic health-care providers serving a diverse population—and where in many cases, they are the only hospitals in a given geographical location—the opt-out clause in the law means a significant number of citizens are deprived of their legal right to physician aid in dying.

Legality of Assisted Dying

The laws we do have legalizing PAD were not created by lawmakers. They owe their passage to grassroots efforts by citizens who have successfully voted them into law. But because few states have an initiative or referendum process enabling citizens to enact laws through the voting process, for the majority of Americans only state or federal legislation can ensure access to legalized PAD.

And even though the only way to ensure equal access across the nation would be through federal legislation, there has never been any federal legislative attempt to legalize physician aid in dying in America.

At the state level, although there have been efforts in some states to introduce bills to the legislature modeled on Oregon's Death with Dignity Act, they have all been unsuccessful to date, although several states are now considering such laws. Our state governments have done little or nothing to assure death with dignity outside of the three states where it is legal.

A telling example of just how forceful the political opposition to PAD has been is demonstrated by the backlash to a legislative effort in California to introduce a law similar to Oregon's Death with Dignity Act. In 2005, where 70 percent of Californians favored passage of the law (California Assembly House Bill 651),[89] the following year the state legislature defeated the bill. The issue has also gone before legislatures in Florida, Hawaii, New Hampshire, Rhode Island, Arizona, and Vermont, and despite public opinion favoring the legalization of physician aid in dying, all these attempts failed.

And where grassroots citizen efforts to legalize PAD succeed, they may be met by forceful efforts to unravel the laws before they are even enacted. Ironically, the prize for a legislature acting against the public will goes to Oregon, the very state that was the first to make physician aid in dying legal. Here's how it happened. In a general election in 1994, the voters of Oregon passed an initiative making physician aid in dying legal. But the opposition succeeded in defying the public will in the Oregon legislature by nullifying the vote under a process allowed in that state. Of interest, in 1997 the Oregon electorate again approved the Death with Dignity Act by a much greater margin than the 1994 vote.

The tense, emotionally charged political and legal battles that have characterized efforts to pass or block legislation regarding PAD have given rise to an important question. Is it a constitutional right to have or engage in physician-assisted dying? And conversely, is banning it protected by our constitution? Because states apply antisuicide laws to PAD to justify prohibiting the practice, the constitutionality of antisuicide laws applies. Yet to date, the question of whether assistance in dying is a constitutionally protected act has reached a state's highest court only once, in Montana, and even there the court sidestepped the broader issue of whether assisted dying is constitutionally protected. In a case testing whether a physician had a right to assist a terminally ill man's "suicide," the Montana Supreme Court ruled that physicians could not be prosecuted for assisted dying, based on current Montana law. But it stopped short of ruling on whether there is constitutional protection for the act.[90]

But there is a federal ruling that allows states to ban PAD. In 1997 the US Supreme Court upheld state laws against assistance in suicide and found they also applied to physician aid in dying. The ruling was the result of concurrent constitutional challenges from two states, Washington and New York, in which plaintiffs alleged that it was unconstitutional to make it a felony for physicians to assist a terminally ill patient to die. Of interest, in both cases, based on liberty and "equal protection" clauses of Fourteenth Amendment, the *federal circuit courts* agreed the antisuicide laws were unconstitutional as applied to physician assistance in dying for terminally ill patients. However, on appeal to the US Supreme Court, the high court struck down the lower court rulings and upheld the antisuicide state laws that banned physician aid in dying.[91]

What was the reasoning behind the court's ruling? First, we must note that the US Supreme Court made no distinction between suicide and physician aid in dying. In the Court's opinion, Chief Justice Rehnquist stated, "The question before the Court is more properly characterized as whether the 'liberty' specially protected by the [due process] Clause [of the 14th amendment] includes a right to commit suicide which itself includes a right to assistance in doing so."[92] In short, the Court considered physician aid in dying as suicide, and so upheld state laws banning assistance in it.

Of course states do have an interest in preserving life, and if that right extends to suicide, assisting the act would indeed violate the presumed state interest. But as we have shown, PAD is not a form of suicide as intended by these laws. When state antisuicide laws were enacted 150 years ago, no one had in mind a dying patient whose life had been medically and artificially extended to an unnatural condition of prolonged suffering. The Oregon and Washington statutes take this historical intent into account and specifically state that physician aid in dying under these laws is *not* suicide. The fundamental conflict these questions illuminate is whether the state's interest ought to be to preserve life at all costs by prolonging it through whatever means necessary, or if the state's interest ought to be promoting the interest of the dying patient.

The real question should be whether the state's interest in preserving life is so absolute as to condemn patients to unnatural, medically managed dying with extended suffering. If so, what might be the implications for physicians who withdraw life-sustaining treatments or administer morphine drips or palliative sedation? Should the state prohibit those acts as well? According to the Supreme Court, those acts, including terminal sedation (see chapter 5)—which invariably lead to unnatural death—are protected. [93]

And just what is the logic by which the court allows terminal sedation but not physician aid in dying? The justices resolved this contradiction by drawing on the issue of *intent*, saying that in physician aid in dying, physicians *intend* to kill their patients, while in palliative sedation they intend to sedate their patients—with death as an "unintended" side effect! They swallowed the fallacious medical excuse hook, line, and sinker.

In defense of its opinion, the court shifted the question from whether it is legal for states to refuse efforts to end life to the assertion that there is a legal *obligation* to *preserve* life. But there is a flaw to this reasoning: if that is the case, shouldn't states mandate maximum curative or life-extending therapy for everyone, right up to the moment of death? The courts have thus far tended to argue that because the state has an interest in preserving life, those interests cannot be undermined by PAD. Yet if the courts genuinely believed the interest in preserving life is so great that PAD should be prohibited, they would find that any failure to preserve life indefinitely is a violation of that interest. But they have thankfully not taken that step because they know it goes too far. If states do not have the right to force patients to prolong their lives through life support, as the US Supreme Court has ruled, why then do they say the state's interest is against allowing suffering patients a right to request physician assistance to end their lives?

These serious questions fall under the broader issue of determining just what constitutes suicide, and asking whether the traditional state interest in preventing suicide applies to patients who otherwise do not want to end their lives but are nonetheless dying. When the term "suicide" is applied to terminally ill patients to justify keeping them alive, their suffering and dying are prolonged. If subjecting someone to unnecessary and extreme suffering is a form of torture, then compelling the terminally ill to unnecessary suffering by labeling PAD as "suicide" is indeed a form of torture.

For terminally ill patients, the state interest in preserving or prolonging life has been met, or more than met, since, with rare exceptions, when a patient with a terminal illness has had medical treatment for the underlying disease, the patient has had his or her life extended or prolonged beyond the point of natural death. The state interest should be to prolong life only so long as doing so doesn't harm the patient, not to prolong life for as long as is technically possible and in the clinician's best interest, not the patient's.

Another state interest cited by the US Supreme Court as a reason for not allowing physician aid in dying is to preserve "the integrity of the medical profession." In *Washington v. Glucksberg*, Chief Justice Rehnquist wrote, "The state also has an interest in protecting the integrity and ethics of the medical profession … Physician-assisted suicide could, it is argued, undermine the trust that is essential to the doctor-patient relationship by blurring the time-honored line between healing and harming."[94]

The chief justice was echoing the language found in the American Medical Association's code of ethics. As we saw in chapter 3, the healing/harming dichotomy the AMA promulgated drew on the Hippocratic teachings that predate Christ and have not been used in any meaningful respect since the nineteenth century. While the spirit of "doing no harm" remains intact, the truth is physicians often and inadvertently "do harm" in their practices every day, through prescribing drugs and other treatments that have adverse consequences to patient health, especially in dying patients, and sometimes by electing not to pursue specific treatment options (often due to the determination of third-party insurers whose refusal to cover certain treatments denies patients any access to treatments that could help or even cure them). Thus the claim that physicians must heal and do no harm is a spurious one predicated on the false dichotomy between healing and curing and on the assumption that medical care is always inherently helpful when, in fact, it is too often fraught with undesirable effects.

In support of this opinion, the chief justice was not only selective in how he cited AMA statements to conform to his opinion, he also disregarded other information and opinions.[95] Of interest, the wishes of patients to forego life-sustaining treatments, an issue prominent in previous decades and in which the court was involved, initially brought resistance from physicians who claimed their integrity would be threatened if they were not allowed to provide all the means at their disposal to save lives.[96] It was the old "healing versus killing argument," and the court got it backward by assuming that keeping a dying patient alive is healing while giving the patient the choice to die is harming.

The court seemed more interested in the opinion of the AMA than the concerns of others, not to mention dying patients, and showed no apparent understanding of how much harm is done by not allowing suffering patients to die.

But why should the highest court in the land so readily support a medical society that speaks for fewer than half the physicians of the country and does not accurately represent even its own members on this issue? I would argue that the court used the expedient of borrowing the AMA's own fallacious rationale to support their personal ideologies and to justify sidestepping a politically sensitive topic. That is, given the rising political clout of a conservative sector of the population that has made abortion a litmus test for partisan politics, any judicial declaration in favor of PAD risks a backlash from this powerful minority that also wants to overturn the landmark *Roe v. Wade* decision granting women the right to abortion. By refusing to acknowledge a constitutional right to PAD, which could potentially strengthen future legal arguments to preserve the right to abortion, the court took the easy way out. And in so doing, it hid behind the AMA's rationale from the Pythagorean-influenced Hippocratic Oath to avoid tackling the thorny issue of whether people have a right to control their own bodies and end their own lives.

Moreover, even if it were argued that the court was not using the AMA's code of ethics to obscure a more politically motivated finding and it truly was concerned with the integrity of the profession, there remains an equally disturbing ramification to such reasoning. While states have a legitimate interest in the well-being of their professions and their practitioners, whose integrity is more important—that of the executive branch of the AMA or of dying patients? Dying patients, not the medical profession, are in need of legal protections. The state interest should first be to serve the public, not the narrower interests of professionals who serve them. Would we ask any less of the legal profession? Should the courts protect the "integrity of the legal profession" above the best interests of the public? To point to the interests of the integrity of the medical profession over the interests of our patients is a profound slap in the face to the patients who entrust their doctors to put patient interests before the interests of the AMA. (That this fallacious argument is presented as a unified voice of the profession is also a slap in the face to physicians, given that the majority of practicing physicians are not members of the association.)

With regard to the court's opinion that helping terminally ill patients die would "undermine the trust that is essential to the doctor-patient relationship by blurring the time-honored line between healing and harming," this statement ignores all other methods by which doctors help their patients die. I would argue that the public is far less likely to lose trust in the medical profession when physicians, at their patients' requests, help them die by turning off ventilators or not resuscitating them than by being told they cannot help them die peacefully because is not in the best interest of their profession.

We should instead ask, "Does the public lose trust in physicians by not helping them die when furthering life beyond the point of natural dying would only prolong suffering?" As Justice Stevens wrote in a dissenting opinion, "For some patients, it would be a physician's refusal to dispense medication to ease their suffering and make their death tolerable and dignified that would be inconsistent with the healing role."[97] Patients increasingly fear their doctors will use technology to keep them alive longer than they wish, rather than fear their doctors will kill them against their wishes, as the court's reasoning implies. Sadly, the court's "physicians must heal, not cure" reasoning is more likely to *undermine* the public's trust in the medical profession because it prolongs the dying process and preempts the comfort care terminally ill patients need.

Furthermore, in reaching its conclusion, the court relied on an opinion unsubstantiated by facts. In a study reported in 1996, 91 percent of patients felt physicians who help their patients die would be as trustworthy to care for critically ill patients as physicians who would not participate in physician aid in dying.[98] Two psychiatrists concluded, "Physician aid in dying will not result in any damage to the medical profession or the public's trust in doctors."[99] Many patients value the willingness of their physicians to discuss physician aid in dying, while a lack of willingness to discuss it impedes openness to discuss other end-of-life issues.

The bottom line is this: some patients who disapprove of physician aid in dying for ideological reasons may distrust physicians who approve of it, while patients who want the option of physician aid in dying may distrust physicians who disapprove of it. And the majority of patients probably wouldn't distrust their physicians either way. But physicians and others who say participation in physician aid in dying would undermine the integrity of the medical profession are stating their own minority view and should not be confused with fact. In the coming years, an unwillingness to participate in or even discuss physician aid in dying is most likely what will undermine the integrity of the medical profession. By politicizing end-of-life care to such an extent that we stop discussing it, our ability to provide that care is undermined. Physicians should put the integrity of their patients, not their professions, first, and by failing to openly and honestly confront the need for PAD, and the manner in which physicians do assist with death through palliative treatment and withdrawal of life support, physicians are failing their patients, their profession, and the public that has entrusted them.

Conclusion

D EATH WITH DIGNITY IS a human right, and in the foregoing pages I have outlined my argument not only for why it ought to be considered a fundamental right of every patient, I have shown the many ways in which that right is denied to the dying. No matter how forcefully a person fights to have help ending their suffering, they may find family members, right-to-life activists, politicians, and even their own doctors going to extremes to prevent a dying person's wish to have his or her suffering end. Just as Hercules's son refused his father's plea to end his agony, so too do those who love us sometimes find it difficult to grant this final wish. Only through laws assuring access to physician-assisted death can we be assured that our wishes, and our wishes alone, will determine how and when we die should our dying be prolonged.

Yet for all the efforts to make such laws a possibility, as of this writing only three states—Oregon, Washington, and Montana— have laws legalizing physician-assisted death. But unfortunately, even under these laws, many dying patients are unable to exercise their right to die because many physicians are unwilling to help their patients in this way and because there remains a powerful movement to obstruct those laws by an ideological minority who are opposed to physician aid in dying. Physicians' denial, deception, and delusion prevents the relief of suffering for many.

How can this happen in a society based on law and religious freedom? It goes without saying there are many civil or secular, nonprofessional and nonreligious reasons to be careful when helping people die by any method. Historically, broad civil injunctions against helping people die have served to prevent true suicide and murder or the killing of people who do not wish to die. Similarly, the principle of sanctity of life is the bedrock of our moral system. But historically, all societies have made exceptions to the rules against the taking of lives, whether for individual or community self-defense, punishment, martyrdom, or to relieve suffering in very special circumstances. However, as should be clear by now, times, circumstances, and needs have changed. Foremost among these changes is our modern medical management of medicalization of dying. The old rules, applied without accounting for the harm they can wreak on today's dying patients, are the source of ever-increasing suffering. We must maintain the utmost caution in changing the rules of how we may help dying patients, but to resist change in the name of doctrine or unfettered custom is to passively promote much suffering with disregard for the values and wishes of others.

Throughout time, all cultures have found that when technologies change, so also do the rules regulating those technologies. Death and dying are no different; with medical technologies changing how and when we die, we must make room for new cultural rules about how we will use these technologies. And that does not mean compelling an entire nation to embrace a singular religious belief system that forces us to endure greater suffering just because we have the technology to keep us alive beyond our natural deaths. It does mean accommodating diverse views about when to use this technology to keep ourselves and our patients alive, and when to use this technology to end suffering and bring life to a more gentle ending.

When cultures clash, how can we fully honor the religious rights of all while preventing individuals, groups, or governments from restricting the legitimate wishes of others? First, we must ask who may be permitted to end a person's life. The answer is clear—only the person whose life is to be ended. No one else may be sanctioned to make the decision or carry out the act of ending a life. Only by this requirement can we be sure it is the patient's reasoned desire, and that others do not engage in euthanasia, or administration of a lethal medication. Abuse can always happen, but with this requirement it is illegal, as at present. We can maintain the timeless secular and religious rules for protecting life by empowering only those individuals whose lives have been artificially altered to a process of slow, tortured dying. Second, among the many who suffer, who may be permitted to end their own life? The answer: only those who through medical management have avoided natural death and are now in a state of prolonged dying with suffering.

And how may patients in a medically induced state of prolonged dying end their lives? It is the duty of those who have changed how their patients die—our medical providers—to help minimize the suffering they have caused at the end of patients' lives. As from the time of Hippocrates, we must turn to the physicians who have cared for us throughout our lives to care for us throughout our deaths, and to do so for the benefit of the patients they serve, not the profession they serve. This is not empowering individuals or a class of persons to violate the old rules. And it is not empowering physicians to kill us. It is allowing physicians to help their patients. It is patients who are empowered through assisted-dying laws, not their physicians.

The Physicians' Choice—Duty or Delusion?

Over the last several decades, physicians and their professional groups have used the slogan, if not mantra, of *patient-centered* medicine. This harkens back to the phrase of the Hippocratic Oath I like best: "Into whatever homes I go, I will enter them for the benefit of the sick." That is, for the benefit of the patient, not someone else and not for the benefit of the physician. What higher purpose and what better reminder could there be for each individual physician, not to mention how the phrase elevates the profession as a whole?

Yet when it comes to helping patients lessen end-of-life suffering, far too many physicians are *not* patient-centered. When they say, "I can't do that," or "That's not my job," they are practicing *physician-centered*, not patient-centered, medicine. If medicine is to be patient-centered, its practitioners must look at their patients and ask, "What do you want? What can I do to help you?"

To say it is not the job of physicians to help their patients die is the great "cop-out" of end-of-life medical care. As we have seen, many physicians always have and clearly do help their patients die when it is the best way to reduce harm. It is delusional to say the modern practices of morphine drips, palliative sedation, and withdrawing life-supporting treatments are not means of helping patients die. Being self-delusional is bad enough, but deceiving the public is worse. Physicians have been helping patients die for as long as medicine has been practiced, yet they remain in the forefront of resisting laws to make it legal to do so because they are uncomfortable with doing so openly and accepting responsibility for the suffering that medical technology can cause.

The physician who says, "We just don't do that," is often saying, "I won't do it because I haven't done it before." Should eighteenth-century physicians have said, "We don't do that" when asked to vaccinate a child? Should a humane physician back away from what he has not before done, or should he determine to *learn* how to help his patient?

Many physicians have said to me, "But I just don't think I can do it. All my training has been to keep my patients alive. This is the opposite—we're not trained to do this." Please, oh please. Are physicians unable to learn new skills? Almost all the procedures and treatments physicians provide for their patients today were unknown just seventy-five years ago—physicians had to learn! And learning patient care is not limited to just learning new biophysical techniques. It also means learning new models of patient care—in other words, learning new ways of viewing the patient/healer relationship and the roles of the physician. It doesn't take a month of study or attendance at a continuing medical education course to write a prescription for a dying patient. What it may take is a new understanding of why writing that prescription is a healing act of the highest standard of patient care. Avoiding doing so is often less about "old dogs" not being able to learn new tricks as it is about the natural proclivity of most physicians to avoid anything socially controversial.

Other physicians say, "Am I now going to have to think about when my patient wants to die, rather than how to keep him alive?" Well, yes. It is a part of patient care. Should this be a surprise? When more and more of all medical care is for patients with terminal illnesses, why should a patient-centered physician resist wanting to learn about treating the inevitable end of all his efforts? Are physicians more willing to abandon their patients than learn how to help them? Sadly, as we have seen, far too many do just that.

Is the unwillingness of physicians to help their dying patients also the result of a medical system geared toward lucrative procedures and not rewarding physicians for time spent listening to and helping with the requests of dying patients? In some real part it is. Physicians are trained to do what pays well and what they like to do, so maybe it's understandable that they resist training for something lacking in both those aspects. But then, what does "patient-centered" mean if not centered on the needs of the patient, not the physician?

For all the debates there have been on the topic of physician-assisted death, there remains a troubling failure on the part of physicians to be honest with the public about the ways in which they do assist the dying. They also fail to be honest with themselves about the topic. Many physicians continue to delude themselves and deceive their patients with a double standard about physician aid in dying. In a survey of about three hundred physicians in 1991, 49 percent favored making physician aid in dying legal, but 75 percent did not want to participate in it. But when asked if they would like the option for themselves, 70 percent said they would like to have it as an option if they were terminally ill. These findings suggest physicians use professional standards and rules of conduct when dealing with their patients but resort to personal beliefs when considering themselves. This is the reverse of the Golden Rule—do unto me as I refuse to do unto others.[100]

There are many professional reasons physicians back away from helping their terminal patients die, but the time has come for physicians to stop the self-delusion about their role and face up to their duty to help their dying patients and not harm them by abandoning them to extended suffering.

Remember the story of how Hercules, in facing great suffering at his end, demands of his son to help him die. When his son said, "You are asking me to be your murderer," Hercules replied, "No, I am not. I ask you to be my healer, the only physician who can cure my suffering." Things have changed little from twenty-five hundred years ago. Sophocles's story encapsulates the conflict between physicians—who want to be healers—and their dying patients who want relief of suffering. Physicians must recognize their duty, and change for the "benefit of the patient," if they are genuinely to embrace patient-centered medicine.

Freedom from Ideological Oppression

As I have shown, for many people, resistance to physician-assisted dying is strongly founded on religious beliefs, and among these, the conservative right-to-life movement has been the most vocal and effective in blocking laws for aid in dying and access to it where it is legal. Given our society's commitment to freedom of religion, how can one faith have such dominance in medical decision making? It is contrary to the very principles of our nation for one group with a particular religious view opposing PAD to effectively prevent many other people, whose faith embraces and accepts PAD, from exercising their legal right to act according to their values. Is free exercise of religion, as stated in the First Amendment to our Constitution, allowed only for those with certain beliefs?

When I was an intern at a major university hospital, I helped care for a woman who had given birth to a baby girl just ten days before but had continued to bleed to the point of being dangerously anemic. Everyone on our medical team thought she should have a blood transfusion immediately, but she refused. I among others told her of the high risk—almost a certainty—of dying without getting blood, and pleaded for her to allow it. But she wouldn't do it, she explained, because it was against her religion to do so. She was a Jehovah's Witness. The next day she died, leaving a newborn baby with no mother.

As you can guess, this was a traumatic experience I have revisited in my mind many times. Should we have forced her to receive a transfusion, perhaps by physically restraining her while doing it? The answer, I'm afraid, is troubling. Compelling a transfusion to save her life might have been moral and humane. But honoring her wishes because she was informed of the risk and it was her decision, based on her deeply held values, was equally moral and humane. It was, in the wording of the First Amendment, honoring her "free exercise" of religion to let her refuse treatment and subsequently die. And in this country, freedom of religion is important. We may argue with the consequence of free exercise of religion in this case, and be saddened about it, but I can only agree with the fundamental precept of freedom of religion and its preeminent place in our legal and moral functioning. So long as it doesn't harm other people, we must allow free expression of religion even when we disagree with specific expressions of it.

This very moral conundrum is why Oregon and Washington's death-with-dignity statutes allow any medical provider to "opt out," under a "conscience" clause, from participating in helping a patient die under the law. To force an individual to act against his religious convictions would be contrary to free exercise of religion. But what about the other side of the coin? Should individuals or groups who oppose an act be allowed to prevent a patient or medical provider whose religion *supports* the act from doing as he sees morally right? This is precisely what is happening when medical facilities and providers' groups owned by ideologically opposed religious groups deny PAD in the states where it is legal, and when minority factions oppose the majority within professional and political systems by pressuring physicians not to legally engage in the practice.

There is a genuine irony to the religious arguments for mandating or prohibiting specific forms of medical care. To many persons of faith or of nonfaith, a defilement of God-given life, or of natural life, is against God's will, or unethical. But suppose a new or established religion formally codified for its members the belief that *using* a feeding tube to artificially maintain life in a patient who is permanently unconscious would be demeaning of sacred life and hence against God's will? Would physicians then be legally obligated to *remove* the feeding tube of such a patient, regardless of the patient's wishes? The very religious freedom that prevents patients from having the option of PAD could just as easily be grounds for allowing PAD if it were framed as the free exercise of religion. But because the far right religious movement has effectively politicized its values, the possibility of other religious or secular viewpoints shaping how we live and die has been hindered, while the minority view of a fundamentalist Christian group has gained ground.

How then should we determine which religious belief is entitled to free exercise? Should a belief be held as invalid, or inferior, if it is not based on a longstanding religious orthodoxy? When the government allows ideological opponents of PAD to prevent others from exercising their religious beliefs supporting PAD, the government is not protecting religious freedom. Quite the contrary; it is giving its endorsement to a dominance of a particular set of religious beliefs.

As critically desirable as freedom of religion is for all of us, it is meaningless unless there is freedom from the religious practices of others. And to those who suggest that in a democracy majority rule means that if a majority holds a particular religious belief, it is legitimate when those beliefs shape our laws, I say nonsense. Imagine if Jehovah's Witnesses became a majority in our country, or had sufficient political leverage to impose their views. Would it be legitimate to prevent the rest of us from getting blood transfusions? Those of us in this country who do not hold to fundamentalist Islamic belief do not want Sharia law imposed on us. Likewise, we do not want fundamentalist Christianity imposed on us if those are not our beliefs. Yet it is an extraordinary convergence of demographic, geographic, political, economic and legal circumstances that allows a minority of citizens in this country to ban PAD for many people, through protection of free exercise of their own fundamentalist religious beliefs. Would Christ's disciples have denied him a quicker end to his suffering if it had been possible?

Too often in end-of-life matters some religious groups confuse the right to *exercise* their religion with a right to *impose* their religion on Americans who don't share it. The history of religion is sadly rife with examples of horrific persecution of believers and nonbelievers alike in the name of religious correctness. Surely the best protection of religious freedom is to allow all to have free exercise of spiritual beliefs within the law, which must include freedom from oppression of other religions.

Nevertheless, valid religious-cultural positions can overlap and compete, creating legal problems in setting boundaries for religious expression. For example, when the Department of Health and Human Services created a religious exemption to its mandate requiring employers to pay for contraception, sterilization, and the days-after pill, the exemption covered only churches and did not include religious hospitals, schools, and charities. Had it included all religious institutions it would have mandated a broad restriction of these services for many people who want them. Yet many opponents of these services see this as a restriction of free exercise of religion, or "defining religious liberty down," and accused the Department of Health and Human Services of "using the levers of power to bend us to your will."[101]

But for a physician, the provision of PAD is as conscience-based as refusal to perform it is conscience-based for physicians who oppose the practice. Whether or not PAD provision is "conscientious" depends on what conscience is. For physicians, most ideas of conscience involve ethical or religious beliefs—"core" moral beliefs.[102]

In this country, such conflicts are bound to occur, and we need to work on good faith, mutually acceptable solutions to such conflicts. But in a nonauthoritarian society, I believe the free exercise of religion should not be allowed to abridge the legal conscientious rights of other citizens.

It is also time we reexamine our meaning of the "sanctity of life." Helping terminally ill people die more peacefully does not mean repudiating respect for or sanctity of life, which remains the most important ethical principle of our legal and medical systems. But we must question the meaning of sanctity of life in the context of extended dying in new, unnatural conditions. The heiress Sunny von Bülow, whose own husband tried to kill her with insulin, was in a coma for nearly twenty-eight years during which doctors said she never showed any signs of brain activity. To sanctify such a wretched, ungodly state of life ultimately harms the principle of sanctity of life itself. We need a public rethinking of how our current rules regarding freedom of religion can work against those whose heartfelt values aren't as protected as the right of a Jehovah's Witness to refuse a blood transfusion or of a Catholic physician to refuse removal of a feeding tube.

Hercules's request and his son's refusal to help him die foretold the dilemma of dying in the twenty-first century. Many physicians today feel inhibited by the crossfire of medical tradition, religious and/or ethical strictures, political and legal hazards, and professional training. But the world has changed mightily. Why should ancient ideology and an intransigent medical tradition continue to increase the suffering of our dying people? All traditions, in all societies, are the stuff of change. Traditions change with changing technologies, with changing times, and changing forms of social organization. Just as slavery was once a valued tradition, and bloodletting an honored medical tradition, those traditions have rightly passed. And with these changing times, we physicians need to change our way of thinking about how our patients die.

Above all, the majority of Americans who support physician aid in dying on grounds of moral value should not remain passive while so many of our friends and relatives face extended dying with agonizing physical and emotional pain, helplessness, and indignity. It is time to make your voices heard—in your physician's office, in your home, and in your community. Do not go silent into that good night if what you ultimately seek is to go gently.

Recommendations

THE FUTURE OF DYING is upon us, with transplants, artificial organs, genetically developed drugs, pacemaker-defibrillators, and much more changing how and when we die. But because of the cultural-religious taboo against helping patients die, patients, families, and physicians all face new dilemmas in choosing which medical treatments to pursue and which to decline.

In the years to come, patients and their physicians will face more and more difficult decisions about ever-more complex therapies that carry some possibility for reasonable extension of life but which also carry the risk that, should they fail, can intensify suffering and prolong dying until life is utterly unbearable. If we don't provide patients the means to relieve that unbearable suffering at the end of life, dying will become all the more complex with even greater suffering. More and more patients will choose to decline what could be beneficial treatments because they fear what might happen if the treatment fails.

As medical technology pushes harder against the margins of life, what patients want is assurance that if they do take a medical risk they won't be stuck in the limbo of extended dying if or when the treatment fails. To gain this assurance they need and ought to be able to have some sort of agreement or directive that allows them to terminate the dying process if treatment is not working.

In fact, such an agreement happened in the highly celebrated case of Barney Clark. When Clark got the world's first implanted artificial heart in 1982, his physicians knew it might not work well enough to sustain any meaningful life. For this reason they gave him a key with which he could turn off the artificial heart if his condition became unbearable. He even had an agreement to this effect in his written and duly transacted consent form. It was the first such contract made before a medical treatment. The surgical team's justification for giving him the choice of continuing or ending life was that the treatment would already have extended his life beyond its natural end, and a patient has a right to end treatment. Unfortunately, he became too weak to use the key and survived until his physicians gave up and turned off the artificial heart.

It is quite possible, if not probable, that within twenty-five years, half or more of all dying patients will have had an implanted prosthetic device, an organ transplant, or genetic therapy that has extended their life. Suspended in the half-cure of artificial life, these patients will need—and will deserve—a socially and legally acceptable means of terminating their dying processes if need be.

Physicians must understand and communicate better the contingent nature of many end-of-life treatments to their patients. Patient and physician alike should ask, "What is the purpose of the treatment?" A reasonable goal would be restoration of health, or at the least recovery to a minimal level of awareness and interaction with loved ones, without an unacceptable burden of suffering. Being alive is not the same as having or enjoying a life. No treatment should have as its ultimate result or purpose merely keeping a body alive unnaturally and indefinitely despite unwanted suffering. Yet that is all too often precisely what happens with some end-of-life treatments.

If both patient and doctor understand in advance the conditional or contingent nature of the treatment, they should have an agreement that, should the treatment fail, the physicians will not insist on maintaining the treatment even if it is essential for life support but can be discontinued, or they will offer aid in dying if the patient so chooses.

How to Avoid Excessive End-of-Life Suffering

It takes planning and some advance work to chart a course to peaceful dying.

Dying Peacefully

- Advance directives
- Living will
- Durable power of attorney
- POLST (physician orders for life-sustaining treatment)
- Enforce end-of-life instructions
- Talk to your doctor
- Talk to your family
- Insist on good comfort care (relief of symptoms, physical and emotional)

Whereas in the past dying was largely unexpected and rarely planned for, today, unfortunately, planning for a peaceful end requires considerable work. To guard against prolonged suffering at the end of life, effective planning must include advance directives, discussion of end-of-life wishes with family and doctors, and an agreement or understanding about use of physician aid in dying if necessary.

Advance Directives

If you want any control over how you die, begin by getting an advance directive. These are the legal documents that outline your desires and goals for how you do and do not want to die.

A *living will* is the best means of making a statement to medical professionals of how aggressively you want to be kept alive with life-prolonging medical care if you should become terminally ill or permanently unconscious and unable to make medical decisions. To prepare your living will (sometimes called a health-care directive), get an approved form from your doctor's office, health-care facility, an advocacy group such as Compassion & Choices, or city, county, or state departments of health.

In your living will, list the conditions under which you would or would not want treatment intended to prolong life. Specify whether you want your directions to apply only if you are terminally ill, or even if you do not have a terminal condition. In case you are not terminally ill, state the conditions under which you would want to be allowed to die, such as unconsciousness or coma from which you probably will not recover; irreversible complete or nearly complete loss of ability to think and communicate; total permanent dependency on others for bodily care; pain that cannot be eliminated, or can be controlled only by sedation so heavy you cannot communicate with others; irreversible dementia such as Alzheimer's disease; and other circumstances in which you would not want life-sustaining treatment (which you must clearly describe).

Give instructions as to which specific treatments you want stopped so they will not keep you alive, such as resuscitation by electrical shock if your heart stops; artificial breathing by a mechanical ventilator; antibiotics for life-threatening infections; feeding (nutrition and hydration) either intravenously or through a tube inserted into your stomach; all medicines to prevent failure of any organ; dialysis for kidney failure; transfusions of blood or other fluids; and anything else intended to keep you alive. A special note: if you have an implanted heart defibrillator designed to shock your heart if it should stop beating effectively, state clearly that you want it turned off under the conditions listed above.

These choices are the heart of your instructions to physicians and family as to when and under what conditions you want treatment to stay alive or you want to avoid treatment that would prolong your life. But alone they aren't enough, as physicians and/or family might decide you would choose differently if you could understand their reasons for keeping you alive, and then act contrary to your stated wishes. To give further legal clout to your desires, a second advance directive is necessary.

A *Durable Power of Attorney* for health care is a means for you to designate someone else to make medical decisions for you if you become unconscious or unable to make decisions. Forms for this advance directive are available from the same places where you can get living will forms (a single form that combines both a living will and a durable power of attorney is available). On this form, you should name an attorney-in-fact, or agent, who will have strong legal standing to make decisions for you. Choose someone for your attorney-in-fact who knows your wishes and will faithfully represent you according to the directives in your living will. Make it clear to other family members that your agent will have final authority to act on your behalf.

Get copies of both your living will and durable power of attorney into the medical records of each medical office you visit and every medical institution (hospital, nursing home, rehabilitation center) where you have been a patient and may possibly return. Give a copy of each to your spouse or partner and to each adult child, as well as to any trusted friend who is likely to be nearby if or when you need these documents. Tell these people to be sure the necessary health-care personnel are aware of your advance directives and have copies, if your condition calls for it.

A newer form of advance directive, called physician orders for life-sustaining treatment (POLST), is a form signed by a physician to express your wishes for care at the end of life. It offers far more detailed options than a simple "do-not-resuscitate" (DNR) directive. An important difference is that the POLST is a type of doctor's orders and cannot be ignored by paramedics or physicians in emergency rooms or anywhere. It is designed to honor patient preferences throughout the health-care system—

including doctor's offices, hospitals, and nursing homes. And it is portable—you can take it with you. Patients who have this type of advance directive are more likely to receive their preferred level of care than patients who use more traditional methods such as advance directives and DNR orders. It is most useful for saying what you do not want, such as resuscitation, a breathing tube, or a feeding tube. Check to see if this newer type of directive is available in your state.

Enforcing End-of-Life Instructions

For all the measures you can and should take to ensure you receive the end-of-life care that you—and not someone else—desires, when it comes to enforcing these directions, you may well discover that your wishes are still difficult to carry out. It is not really enough to just give your doctor your advance directive and hope he or she will abide by them. Many doctors never read a patient's advance directive thoroughly, and some don't even remember which patients have them. Talking to your doctor about your end-of-life wishes and plans can be the critical step to succeeding. It takes your wishes beyond some papers stuffed in the back of your medical chart and humanizes your feelings. Even if your doctor doesn't agree with your way of dying, listening to you talk about it adds a strong dose of sincerity and earnestness to your wishes and could be instrumental in helping your physician treat you according to *your* wishes, not his or hers. Talking to them also helps you understand your doctor(s) and their feelings about your directives and, in case your doctor objects to your plans, it gives you the opportunity to find someone else more empathetic. Patients who have full and open discussions with their doctors about end-of-life wishes are much more likely to die peacefully and can avoid extended agony for their families.

In a study published in the Journal of the American Medical Association in October 2008, Boston researchers found that patients who had end-of-life discussions with their physicians "were more likely to accept that their illness was terminal, prefer medical treatment focused on relieving pain and discomfort over life-extending therapies, and have completed a do-not-resuscitate order."[103] So have that discussion with your doctor, but don't wait until you can hardly breathe out the words. Do it when you deliver your advance directive—it could be years before you need it, but it's never too soon to let your doctor know your feelings and how you want to die. In addition, you can write a letter to your doctor in which you give your general approach to end-of-life issues, how you view dying, and even your spiritual values. It's a bit more personal and meaningful than a legal document. And finally—when you do talk to your doctor, have someone else along with you, a relative or close friend who can help your remember how the conversation went. The other person also serves as a witness who confirms your statements to the doctor and can testify to your final wishes should it become necessary.

Although the majority of people wish to die at home, it is estimated that up to 60 percent of chronically ill patients die in hospitals, and 20 percent die in nursing homes.[104] If you want to die at home and avoid spending the last days or weeks of your life in a medical facility, be sure your physician understands your wishes. And if you're in a nursing home, beware of being sent to a hospital where you may get undesired treatment, spend the rest of your life in an intensive care unit, and lose control of how you die.

Despite all these measures, talking to your family may well be the best means of ensuring the peaceful dying you seek. Unless you have no family and are a hermit, you will not go through the dying process alone. You will need the help of those around you—your family, close friends, and trusted advisors—to support and help you steer your course through the treacherous rapids of medical decision making. As you become less able to speak for yourself, medical providers and caregivers will look more and more to those around you for the important decisions about how you wish to die. This is why your loved ones must know your wishes well in advance of when they will be called upon to help you.

In this day and age, there's no reason you shouldn't sit down with your family as soon as your children are old enough to understand and process your thinking about how—at some time in the distant future—you want to die—and more to the point, how you do *not* want to die. Tell them your feelings and thinking on the subject. A good way to do this is to have a "family planning" discussion, combining discussion of how you intend to handle finances in the future with discussion of how you want to handle medical decisions if or when you should become terminally ill. Use your financial will and your living will as instruments for discussion.

If you do become terminally ill, and after careful and informed consideration of all treatment options and their chances for some meaningful recovery you reach the point of wishing no further prolongation of the dying process, you must let your family know of your readiness to die. Remember, they may not understand your condition or share your decision to let go, especially if you have not prepared them in advance by making clear your choices. But they need to know your feelings and wishes if they are going to be able to help you.

But be prepared. If you are dying, regardless of how well prepared they are, your family will not want to lose you, and one or more of them may do anything possible to avoid facing this reality. If they don't understand or agree with your end-of-life wishes, the best way they know of helping you in your battle against dying is to do anything and everything possible to keep you alive. Remember, your passing away is a loss for those who love you, and they need time to grieve before you go. What often haunts family after a loved one has died is the feeling of guilt over having done "too little" when there was a chance to help.

If you are to resist what may become incessant and persuasive pleas for further attempts at a cure, you must share with them your reasons and determination to let go, if this is your decision.

Until they have worked through the grieving process, they will do everything possible to not let you go. In my experience, this grieving time before a loved one is willing to "let go" is two to six months from the moment of learning a loved one is terminally ill and dying. If you give your loved ones enough time to consider your wishes for end-of-life care, most often they will give you the support you need. Part of the grieving process for them is accepting the inevitability of your dying, a necessary step before they are able to help you reach your goals for peaceful dying. I have worked with many dying patients who had loved ones initially adamantly oppose physician aid in dying but later transformed their feelings to supporting, or at least acquiescing in the terminally ill patient's desire for physician aid in dying. "I wish he wouldn't do it," or "I'm against it," they will say. "But I love him, and it's what he wants to do, so I will support him in his wish."

However, in many cases, the family member or friend who opposes a patient's desire for PAD does so for deeply held ideological reasons. Some of these persons will relent and not oppose the patient's wish after grieving and listening to the plea of the dying patient, but often they will not relent. There are no data on this point, but most certainly a lot of patients who would prefer to die peacefully with PAD never get the chance because of a resolutely opposed spouse or child. I observed a case in which a right-to-life son blocked all his father's attempts to have PAD. In desperation, the dying patient decided to stop eating and drinking, a process that usually takes days before the patient dies of dehydration, as in "palliative sedation." The family and caretakers stopped all liquids and foods and the patient became disoriented, but unbeknownst to other family members, the son stayed with his father through the night for several weeks. Whenever the father woke or stirred, the son gave him enough liquids to keep him alive until he finally died from overwhelming effects of his terminal disease. The son's acts may have been intended to alleviate his father's suffering from starvation and dehydration, but they instead caused immense additional suffering for the dying man and all others in the family.

I reluctantly advise my patients that if they have a relative or relatives who strongly disagree with their plan to die by stopping life-sustaining treatment or by PAD, it is probably better not to tell them about end-of-life plans. This sounds harsh, but in reality, a family member who opposes your plan will in all likelihood prevent you from carrying out your wish, regardless of how many others support your wish. And if you succeed despite the opposition, and he discovers what happened, he may well create more mischief—by going to the police or the local media—than you or your other supportive loved ones would want. Again, giving close family members time to grieve and think through priorities may allow even the most resistant loved one to relent and support you, but it takes time, and those who are fervently opposed usually do not relent. But the more you can prepare for end-of-life care with your family, the greater your chances of a more peaceful dying.

Insist on Good Comfort Care

Above all, insist on good comfort care at your life's end. There is no excuse today for any dying person to be denied adequate comfort care, although it happens for several reasons. Although health-care finances are beyond the scope of this book, suffice to say that some patients do not get good comfort care because they have no means to access it, privately or through public means. With these exceptions, everyone has access to comfort care and should firmly insist on getting it. But as I've shown, even with medical attention and hospice care, too many patients are denied this access.

By protecting your legal rights, however limited they may currently be, with an advance directive and durable power of attorney, and communicating your wishes with your family and health-care providers, you may not be guaranteed the peaceful end you seek, but you will certainly have empowered yourself to make such an end a real possibility once those final days do come.

Notes

1. Denis Demonpion and Léger Laurent, *Le Dernier Tabou, Révélations sur la Santé des Présidents* (Hamilton, MT: Pygmalion Press, 2012).

2. Michael Paterniti, "The Last Meal," *Esquire*, May 1, 1998, www.esquire.com/features/The-Last-Meal-0598.

3. Denis Demonpion and Léger Laurent, *Le Dernier Tabou, Révélations sur la Santé des Présidents* (Hamilton, MT: Pygmalion Press, 2012).

4. The Harris Poll #9, January 25, 2011, available online at http://www.harrisinteractive.com/NewsRoom/HarrisPolls/tabid/447/mid/1508/articleId/677/ctl/ReadCustom percent20Default/Default.aspx.

5. Edith Hamilton, *The Greek Way* (New York: W. W. Norton & Co., 1993): 158.

6. Aeschylus, *Agamemnon*, lines 1448–51.

7. Moses Hadas, *The Stoic Philosophy of Seneca: Essays and Letters* (New York: W. W. Norton & Co., 1986): 202–3.

8. Joseph V. Sullivan, *Catholic Teaching on the Morality of Euthanasia* (Washington: Catholic University of America Press, 1949).

9. Thomas E. Keys, *The History of Surgical Anesthesia* (Park Ridge, IL: Wood Library-Museum of Anesthesiology, 1996): 32–35.

10. President's Council on Bioethics, *Being Human: Readings from the President's Council on Bioethics* (Washington, DC: Government Printing Office, 2003), available online at http://www.bioethics. gov.

11. http://www.catholicnewsagency.com/news/cardinal-burke-suffering-does-not-rid-life-of-purpose/.

12. Ravi Nessman, "Karen Ann Quinlan's Parents Reflect on Painful Decision Twenty Years Later," *Los Angeles Times*, April 7, 1996.

13. Annette E. Clark, "The Right to Die: The Broken Road from Quinlan to Schiavo" (*Loyola University Chicago Law Journal*, 37:383–403, 2006).

14. Joseph and Julia Quinlan, *Karen Ann: The Quinlans Tell Their Story* (New York: Bantam Books, 1978).

15. Margot Dougherty and Sandra Rubin Tessler, "Tiring of Life Without Freedom, Quadriplegic David Rivlin Chooses to Die Among Friends," *People* 32:6, August 7, 1989.

16. Ibid.

17. Marilyn Webb, *The Good Death: The New American Search to Reshape the End of Life* (New York: Random House and Bantam Books, 1999).

18. Kirk Cheyfitz, "Suicide Machine Part I: Kevorkian Rushes to Fulfill his Client's Wishes to Die," *Detroit Free Press*, March 3, 1997.

19. Lori A. Roscoe, L. J. Dragovic, and Donna Cohen, "Dr. Jack Kevorkian and Cases of Euthanasia in Oakland County, Michigan, 1990–98," *New England Journal of Medicine* 343 (December 7, 2000): 1735–36.

20. "Depressed? Don't Go See Dr. Kevorkian," *New York Times*, September 16, 1995.

21. Ibid.

22. Mike Allen, "Counsel to GOP Senator Wrote Memo on Schiavo," *Washington Post*, April 7, 2005.

23. Leon R. Kass, "Why Doctors Must Not Kill," *Commonweal, Special Supplement*, August 2011 (New York, 1991), 14:472–76.

24. Ibid.

25. Statement on euthanasia of the Christian Medical and Dental Associations, available online at http://www.cmda.org/wcm /CMDA/Issues2/End_of_Life1/Assisted_Suicde_Euthanasia /Ethics_Statements4/Physician_Assisted_S.aspx, 2012.

26. The Qur'an states that "tablets" were given to Moses, without quoting their contents explicitly.

27. http://www.catholiceducation.org/articles/politics/pg0029.

28. Augustine, *Concerning the City of God against the Pagans*, bk 1, chap. 21, ed. David Knowles; trans. Henry Bettenson (Harmondsworth: Penguin, 1972).

29. "Charlie," a term used to refer to the North Vietnamese soldiers during the war in Vietnam, was an exception in using a human name to refer to the enemy.

30. The Wedge Document, Discovery Institute, 1999; Phillip E. Johnson, *Defeating Darwinism by Opening Minds* (Downers Grove, IL: InterVarsity Press, 1997): 91–92.

31. Wesley J. Smith, *Discovery Institute News* (June 20, 2006): 7:3–13.

32. *Taking Care, Ethical Caregiving in Our Aging Society*, The President's Council on Bioethics (Washington, DC: September 2005).

33. Ibid., 122.

34. Ibid., 229.

35. WSMA media release, July 2, 2008; Carol Ostrom, "Doctors Divided on Assisted Suicide," *Seattle Times* (Sept 22, 2008): B1:2.

36. Ibid.

37. R. J. McMurray, O. W. Clark, and J. A. Barrasso, "Decisions Near the End of Life," *JAMA* 267 (1992): 2229, 2233.

38. Simon N. Whitney, Byron W. Brown, Howard Brody, Kirsten H. Alcser, et al., "Views of United States Physicians and Members of the American Medical Association House of Delegates on Physician-Assisted Suicide," *J Gen Internal Medicine* 16 (2001): 290–96.

39. Thomas Aquinas, *Summa Theologiae*, 2a2ae64.5 (Blackfriars; New York: McGraw-Hill; London: Eyre & Spottiswoode, 1964).

40. Margaret P. Battin, *Least Worst Death* (Oxford University Press, 1994): 210.

41. It is because the word "suicide" has come to be associated with "killing" that many survivors of suicide persons reject the term "committed suicide"—which focuses on the act—and use instead the term "died from suicide" to emphasize the tragedy and loss.

42. Margaret P. Battin, *Least Worst Death* (Oxford University Press, 1994): 214.

43. http://plato.stanford.edu/entries/suicide/#ChrPro.

44. Margaret P. Battin, *Least Worst Death* (Oxford University Press, 1994): 261.

45. Sacred Congregation for the Doctrine of the Faith: Declaration on Euthanasia. I. "The Value of Human Life." Part 3 (1980). See http://www.priestsforlife.org/magisterium/iuraetbona.htm#valuelife.

46. David Hume, *Essays on Suicide and the Immortality of the Soul* (1783).

47. Arthur Schopenhauer, *Parerga and Paralipomena*, trans. E. F. J. Payne (Oxford: Clarendon Press, 2000).

48. American Medical Association, *Code of Medical Ethics*, Opinion 2.211, issued June 1994 based on the reports *Decisions Near the End of Life*, adopted June 1991, and *Physician-Assisted Suicide*, adopted December 1993 (*JAMA* 1992; 267:2229–33); updated June 1996. Available online at http://www.ama-assn.org/ama/pub/physician-resources/medical-ethics/code-medical-ethics/opinion2211.

49. Thomas A. Preston, *Patient-Directed Dying* (Bloomington, IN: iUniverse, 2006): 23–25.

50. Linda Ganzini, et al., "Mental Health Outcomes of Family Members of Oregonians Who Request Physician Aid in Dying," *Journal of Pain Symptom Management* 38, no. 6 (December 2009): 807–15.

51. Washington State Psychological Association Policy on value-neutral language regarding end-of-life choices, available online at www.wapsych.org, January 8, 2007.

52. Darrel W. Amundsen, *Medicine, Society, and Faith in the Ancient and Medieval Worlds* (Baltimore and London: Johns Hopkins University Press, 1996): 39.

53. Owsei Tempkin, *Hippocrates in a World of Pagans and Christians* (Baltimore and London: Johns Hopkins University Press, 1991): 247.

54. Ibid., 22.

55. *The Art*, 3; cf. *Diseases* 2, 48. See: Darrel W. Amundsen, "The Physician's Obligation to Prolong Life: A Medical Duty without Classical Roots," *Hastings Center Report* (August 1978): 24.

56. National Catholic Bioethics Center, available online at http://www.stgiannaphysicians.org/enshrinements/the-st-gianna-pnysicians-guild-catholic-hippocratic-oath.html.

57. http://www.wma.net/en/30publications/10policies/g1/index.html.

58. Emphasis added.

59. Louis Lasagna, *Life, Death, and the Doctor* (New York: Alfred A. Knopf, 1968): 243.

60. Arthur Kleinman, *Patients and Healers in the Context of Culture: An Exploration of the Borderland between Anthropology, Medicine, and Psychiatry* (Berkeley: University of California Press, 1980).

61. Lewis M. Cohen, *No Good Deed* (New York: HarperCollins, 2010): 56.

62. Edmund D. Pelligrino, "Doctors Must Not Kill," *Journal of Clinical Ethics* 3, no. 2 (1992): 95–102.

63. Jennifer W. Mack, et al., "End-of-Life Care Discussions among Patients with Advanced Cancer: A Cohort Study," *Annals of Internal Medicine* 156 (February 7, 2012): 1–34.

64. Perhaps even more disturbing, it was later concluded that the consent form he signed was very confusing, the procedure not adequately tested on animals prior to implanting in a human, the surgical team inexperienced and inadequate, and the entire procedure "fundamentally unethical." Renee C. Fox and Judith P. Swazey, *Spare Parts: Organ Replacement in American Society* (New York: Oxford University Press, 1992): 102–4.

65. Thomas A. Preston, *Patient-Directed Dying: A Call for Legalized Aid in Dying for the Terminally Ill* (Bloomington, IN: iUniverse, 2006).

66. Address of John Paul II to the Participants in the International Congress on "Life-Sustaining Treatments and Vegetative State: Scientific Advances and Ethical Dilemmas," (20 March 2004). See: http://www.vatican.va/holy_father/john_paul_ii/speeches/2004/march/documents/hf_jp-ii_spe_20040320_congress-fiamc_en.html.

67. http://zocalopublicsquare.org/thepublicsquare/2011/11/30/how-doctors-die/read/nexus.

68. "Decisions Near the End of Life," Council on Ethical and Judicial Affairs, American Medical Association, *JAMA* 267, no. 16 (April 22/29, 1992): 2229.

69. President's Commission for the Study of Ethical Problems in Medicine and Biomedical and Behavioral Research, *Deciding to Forego Life-Sustaining Treatment* (March 1983), 238–39.

70. *Cruzan v. Director, Missouri Department of Health*, 88–1503, 497 U.S. 261, 267–68 (1990).

71. Pius XII, Address of February 24, 1957, *AAS* 49 (1957): 147.

72. Thomas A. Preston, "Professional Norms and Physician Attitudes Toward Euthanasia," *Journal of Law, Medicine & Ethics* 22, no. 1 (Spring 1994): 36–40.

73. Candace Cummins Gauthier, "Active Voluntary Euthanasia, Terminal Sedation, and Assisted Suicide," *Journal of Clinical Ethics*, 12, no. 1 (Spring 2001).

74. Margaret P. Battin, "Terminal Sedation: Pulling the Sheet over Our Eyes," *Hastings Center Report* 38, no. 5 (2008): 27–30.

75. Rob McStay, "Terminal Sedation: Palliative Care for Intractable Pain, Post *Glucksberg* and *Quill*," *American Journal of Law and Medicine*, 29:45–76 (2003).

76. D. Orentlicher, "The Supreme Court and Terminal Sedation: Rejecting Assisted Suicide, Embracing Euthanasia," *Hastings Constitutional Law Quarterly* 24, no. 4 (1997): 947–68.

77. Margaret P. Battin, "Terminal Sedation: Pulling the Sheet over Our Eyes," *Hastings Center Report*, 38:5 (September–October 2008): 27–30.

78. Daniel P. Sulmasy, "Killing and Allowing to Die," *Journal of Law, Medicine & Ethics* 26, no. 1 (Spring 1998): 55–64.

79. Thomas A. Preston, *The Clay Pedestal* (Seattle: Madronna Publishers, 1981): 144.

80. Sherwin Nuland, *How We Die* (New York: Alfred A. Knopf, 1994): 265.

81. Rhonda Byrne, *The Secret* (New York: Atria Books, 2006): 134.

82 Beverly Smith, "Cradled between Heaven and Earth," *J Palliative Care* 25, no. 4 (2009): 294–96.

83. Lynne P. Taylor, "Viewpoint: Can We Really Prepare for Enabling 'Death with Dignity'?" *Neurology Today* 11, no. 13 (July 7, 2011): 6.

84. http://news.health.com/2011/11/17/cancer-doctors-still-not-great-with-patients-pain, "Medical Oncologists' Attitudes and Practice in Cancer Pain Management: A National Survey," *J Clin Oncol* (10.1200/JCO.2011.35.0561).

85. Available online at http://www.nhpco.org/i4a/pages/index.cfm?pageid=5847.

86. Available online at http://zocalopublicsquare.org/thepublicsquare/2011/11/30/how-doctors-die/read/nexus/.

87. Courtney S. Campbell and Jessica C. Cox, "Hospice and Physician-Assisted Death," *Hastings Center Report* (Sept–Oct 2010): 26–35.

88. L. Ganzini, H. D. Nelson, T. A. Schmidt, et al., "Physicians' Experiences with the Oregon Death with Dignity Act," *New Eng J of Med* 342, no. 8 (2000): 557–63.

89. Kathryn L. Tucker and Paul V. O'Donnell, "At the Very End of Life, Empowering Terminally Ill Cancer Patients with the Option of Aid in Dying," *Oncology Issues* (Nov/Dec 2009): 8, 9; M. Field, Field Research Corp., Release #2188; March 15, 2006. Available online at http://www.!eld.com/!eldpollonline/subscribers/RLS2188.pdf. Last accessed Aug. 11, 2009.

90. Kirk Johnson, "Montana Ruling Bolsters Doctor-Assisted Suicide," *New York Times*, December 31, 2009, http://www.nytimes.com/2010/01/01/us/01suicide.html.

91. *Washington v. Glucksberg*, No. 96–110, 1997, US LEXIS, 4039, June 26, 1997.

92. *Supreme Court of the United States*, No. 96–110, syllabus, 18.

93. *Washington v. Glucksberg*, No. 96–110, 1997, US LEXIS, 4039, June 26, 1997.

94. Ibid.

95. Supreme Court of the United States, No. 95–1858, June 26, 1997; see *American Medical Association, Code of Ethics*, 2.211 Council on Ethical and Judicial Affairs, *JAMA*, 267 (1994): 2229–33.

96. Sarah E. Shannon, "Medical Futility and Professional Integrity, Religious Tolerance, and Social Justice," *ASBH Exchange* (Spring: 5, 2006): 10.

97. Supreme Court of the United States, Nos. 96–110 and 95–1858, June 26, 1997.

98. M. A. Graber, B. I. Levy, R. F. Weir, and R. A. Oppliger, "Patients' Views about Physician Participation in Assisted Suicide and Euthanasia," *J Gen Int Med* 11 (1996): 71.

99. David M. Smith and David Pollack, "A Psychiatric Defense of Aid in Dying," *Community Mental Health Journal* 34, no. 6 (1998): 547–56.

100. T. A. Preston, "Professional Norms and Physician Attitudes toward Euthanasia," *Journal of Law, Medicine & Ethics* 22, no. 1 (1994): 37–40.

101. Ross Douthat, "Defining Religious Liberty Down," *New York Times*, July 28, 2012.

102. Lisa H. Harris, "Recognizing Conscience in Abortion Provision," *N Engl J Med* 367 (Sept 13, 2012): 981–83.

103. Alexi A. Wright, Zhang Baohui, Alaka Ray, et al., "Associations Between End-of-Life Discussions, Patient Mental Health, Medical Care Near Death, and Caregiver Bereavement Adjustment," *JAMA* 300, no. 14 (2008): 1665–73.

104. http://www.fiercehealthcare.com/story/end-life-wishes-not -addressed-overused-palliative-care-experts-say/2011-08-01.

INDEX